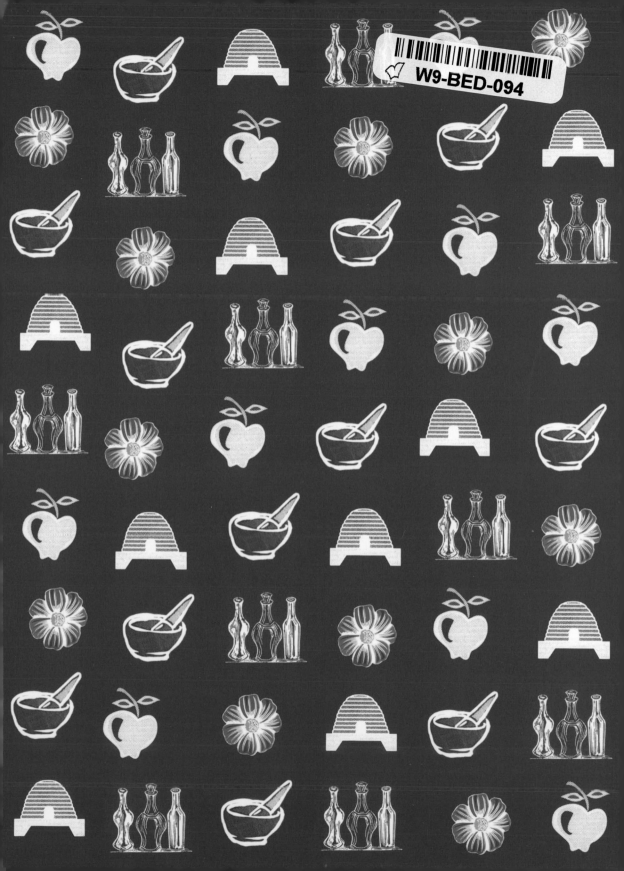

good health magic

good health magic

gill farrer-halls

back-to-basics
Home Remedies
in a flash

MQP

Published by **MQ Publications Limited**

12 The Ivories

6-8 Northampton Street

London N1 2HY

Tel: +44 (0)20 7359 2244

Fax: +44 (0)20 7359 1616

email: mail@mqpublications.com

website: www.mqpublications.com

Copyright © MQ Publications Limited 2003

Text copyright © Gill Farrer-Halls 2003

EDITOR: **Lesley Wilson**

DESIGN: **Balley Design Associates**

ILLUSTRATED BY: **John Fowler, gerardgraphics.co.uk**

ISBN: 1-84072-451-X

1 2 3 4 5 6 7 8 9

Printed and bound in China

Contents

Many people today are seeking natural methods and products to promote good health, tranquility, and beauty. Their search often draws them to the natural herbal remedies of the past, practiced by previous generations. Perhaps they remember a soothing steam inhalation made with herbs during a childhood cold, or they recall rubbing dock leaves on nettle stings and discovering how this magically took away the pain. Such memories provide a powerful stimulus to investigate further the healing power of plants, and to find ways to use them easily in keeping with a modern lifestyle, lived at a faster pace than during our parents' and grandparents' time.

Until the middle of 20th century many households kept a home herbal. This was referred to almost daily for advice, and remedies for everything from minor ailments to beauty tips, from nutritional guidance to perfuming the home. The

Good health—there's got to be a better way!

ingredients suggested in the traditional home herbal were safe, natural, and based on plants. These were grown in the garden or on the windowsill, or were easily available from the local drug store, or village wise woman. Unfortunately with the rise of modern allopathic medicine, much of our grandmothers' ancient herbal lore has been lost. However, now that we are discovering the limitations and disadvantages of antibiotics and other modern medicines, interest in natural remedies is becoming widespread.

Good Health Magic is the modern home herbal. Based on ancient herbal lore, the book incorporates contemporary ingredients and new ideas well suited to our modern, hectic lifestyles. All the remedies and suggestions have natural plant-based ingredients and simple instructions for safety, ease, and convenience. Some of the suggested remedies can be bought ready-made from health food stores and herbal suppliers. Others are quick and easy to make, and give a glimpse of how the wise women and witches used to practice their healing arts.

Good Health Magic also helps you to develop the empowering sense of taking responsibility for your own health. By investigating how you feel and what you need to promote personal health, you naturally take charge of healing your minor ailments and discomforts. Looking at your skin regularly and then working out which herbal treatments are best suited to you at the time keeps you in touch with yourself. Meditation, yoga, tai chi, and self-massage all deepen your connection with your inner being. This relates with the outer environment, which can be made more harmonious by using feng shui. In this way the book embraces different cultural traditions of healing from around the world to promote health and peace, beauty and well-being.

Good Health Magic is an exciting voyage of discovery into the world of plants and learning how to unlock their healing potential. If at first you only dip in briefly and experiment with one or two simple remedies, the healing magic of plants may well draw you in further to try out more. Sometimes it is hard to believe that something so simple as a few stewed herbs can make you feel better—until you try it out for yourself and see.

chapter 1

The Healing Power of Plants

Can a Plant Keep me Healthy?

Of course plants can keep you healthy—healthy and active, whether you're feeling out of sorts or not. It might seem like double Dutch initially, but the more you know about using plants the more you will know what will work for you.

All manner of plants, especially herbs, have been used to promote health and well-being for centuries, throughout the world. Before the rise of allopathic medicine, commonly known as orthodox medicine, herbal remedies played a major role in health care. Whereas herbal medicine uses the natural healing qualities of the whole plant, allopathic medicine relies on the active ingredients of plants isolated in laboratories; these are then sometimes combined with inorganic and synthetic ingredients. This new direction in health care turned its back on the traditional holistic approach of herbal wisdom, which used the whole plant to treat the whole person, rather than a few active ingredients being used to alleviate or suppress the symptoms of a disease.

As a result of the increasing dominance

Naturally, Mother!

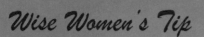

Wise Women's Tip

Many of the traditional herbal healers were the wise women, living in villages, who commanded great respect—and not a little fear—because of their healing powers. The rise of allopathic medicine and its use of inorganic chemicals was accompanied by the systematic disparagement of women's powers to heal using natural herbs and other plants. During the 17th century many women were ultimately condemned as witches, tried by mob, and burned at the stake or drowned, for practising natural herbal medicine.

That's all behind us now, thankfully. Although a certain stigma is attached to alternative medicine, and those who practice it, traditional remedies from Western culture and beyond are becoming increasingly accepted as valuable by the mainstream practitioners of our health services.

of the new allopathic medicine, much of the ancient wisdom of herbal medicine was lost. However, in the past few decades there has been a renewed interest in once again using the power of plants to maintain health and treat disease. This is at least partly because the limitations and side effects of allopathic medicine have become all too obvious, but also because a growing number of people believe in the efficacy of the traditional herbal holistic approach. Many of these people have a desire too, to take some active responsibility for their own health and well-being, without always having to depend on their doctor to treat minor ailments.

A holistic health system

Of course, the value of allopathic medicine needs to be given credit for the progress it has made in health care. In a truly holistic

system allopathic medicine takes its rightful place alongside herbalism, acupuncture, homeopathy, aromatherapy, and all other tried-and-tested treatments available. However, natural methods of healing have been helping people to find health and well-being for much longer than orthodox allopathic medicine. Acupuncture, for instance, is reputed to have existed in China for centuries, while herbal medicine is probably the very oldest of all forms of medicine practised in ancient civilizations thousands of years ago.

In olden days—from medieval times to the early years of the 20th century—every housewife kept a simple home herbal with a variety of remedies, usually plant-based, to cure everyday aches and pains, colds, and injuries due to minor accidents. Wise women healers and doctors were consulted only on occasions when the home herbal proved insufficient for curing the patient. *Good Health Magic* constitutes a modern counterpart to the traditional home herbal, suggesting simple, mostly plant-based remedies to cure common ailments, together with tips on actively promoting health, beauty, and well-being. It certainly does not offer cures for serious illnesses. Always consult a doctor or qualified medical herbalist immediately in cases of serious illness.

In this chapter you will find an introduction to some of the most common and useful herbs, most of which have been safely and successfully used for centuries. Today there are also other plant-based and natural products available that can be used alongside, or instead of, herbs. The most important of these are essential oils: distilled from plants and containing the "essence" or essential nature of the plant. Bach Flower Remedies are simple preparations of flower petals, most of which are prepared by floating the petals on top of spring water in a glass bowl, and leaving this in the sunshine for three or four hours. The resulting flower essences are then boiled in water with a little brandy to preserve them. Bach Flower Remedies are bought ready-prepared but you will learn the most effective way to use the remedies.

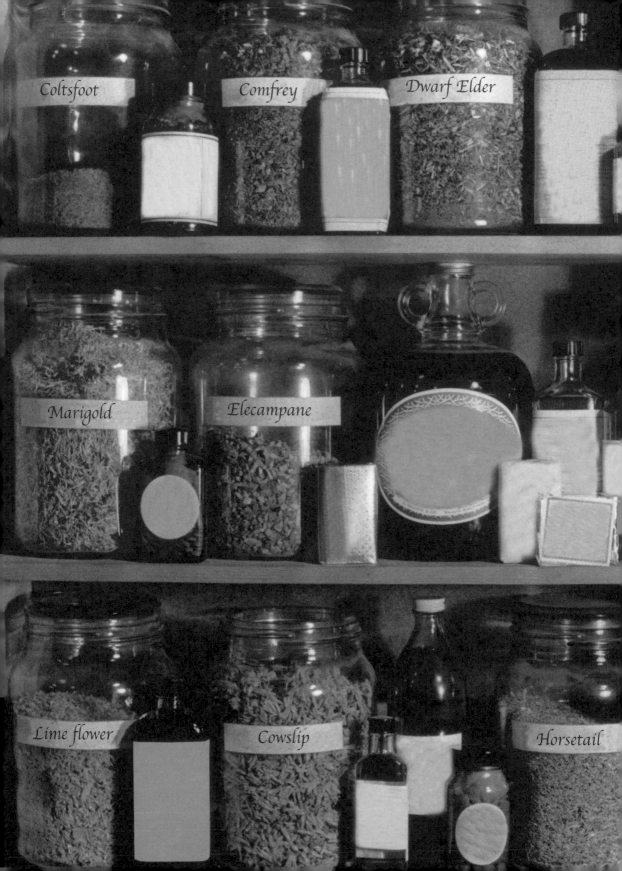

Herbs

Today we are rediscovering the delights of flavoring our food with herbs. But did you know that these herbs—that are easy to buy in the local store or grow on a windowsill—can be used to keep us healthy? You may already enjoy the restorative properties of well-known herbal teas such as peppermint and chamomile but there are many more that you probably don't know about.

Herbal medicine works on the principle of holism, which means that all treatment is based on recognizing every human as a unique life form. Human beings are enlivened by a natural life force, and when some imbalance in this force occurs, illness is experienced. The correct herbs will restore balance to the natural life force, bringing back full health.

This contrasts with the allopathic model, which prescribes a remedy that treats only the person's symptoms, not the underlying imbalance. The holistic approach leads naturally to the idea of preventive medicine, or using herbs to strengthen specific body systems or organs to prevent problems from arising in the first place. So if a tendency to illness or a weakness in the body is present, specific herbs can be taken to reduce susceptibility or strengthen the affected part. In this way some illnesses and diseases can be stopped from developing.

Many herbs can be taken freely without our thinking of them as medicine. Most of us already ingest herbs in some form even if we remain largely unaware of how they help to keep us healthy. Herbs are used extensively in traditional European and Asian dishes to provide flavour. The fact that they benefit the body is an added bonus. Using herbs together with other natural, organic foods to create a balanced, healthy diet is a good way of looking after ourselves. By not loading the body down with additives, chemicals, and artificial preservatives (so-called e-numbers), we have a better chance of staying healthy longer.

Starting to use herbal remedies can be as simple as including garlic, rosemary, oregano, cloves, your diet. Herbal teas are another easy way to ingest the healing power of herbs. These are already in such common use that increasingly sophisticated varieties of herbal teas can be easily found in supermarkets, as well as in health food stores. Listed below is a selection of traditional herbs that are easy to find, and that have been used safely and to

Herbal Lore

In Medieval times, evil spirits were blamed for illness. Perhaps garlic's reputation for warding off vampires and the evil eye springs from its ability to rid people of various ailments.

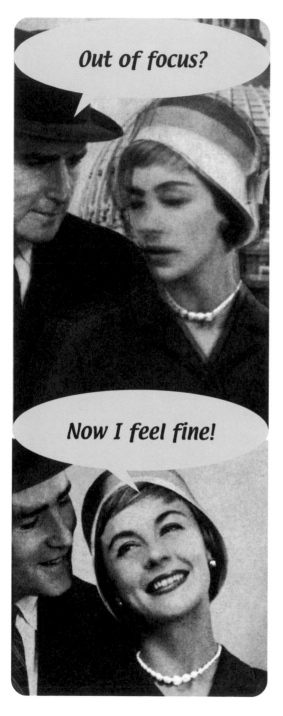

great effect for generations. The common name is given together with the botanical name, as both are used in labeling by shops and suppliers of herbs. The common name often gives an indication of what the herb might be used for, though sometimes the name might seem a little quaint or obscure.

Chamomile—both **Roman Chamomile** (*Chamaemelum nobile*) and **German Chamomile (*Matricaria recutita*)**: Both are in common use. Chamomile was called "maythen" by the Saxons and was one of nine sacred herbs. It was used with other herbs and mixed with rushes for "strewing" floors in the Middle Ages. Chamomile treats a long list of ailments but it is primarily used to ease insomnia, indigestion, and inflammation and to induce relaxation. Avoid during pregnancy.

Comfrey (*Symphytum officinale*): Comfrey has a long history of use in traditional herbal medicine, especially for healing wounds, fractures, and sprains. Comfrey contains allantonin, a naturally occurring chemical that stimulates cell proliferation and regeneration. It is used mainly to promote the healing of external wounds and proper development of scar tissue.

Dandelion (*Taraxacum officinale*): This common garden weed might be the enemy of gardeners, but is in fact a useful herbal remedy. Dandelion is a powerful and valuable diuretic. Because dandelion contains potassium, it prevents the loss of this vital chemical from the body, whereas other diuretics can cause loss of potassium. Dandelion is also a good general tonic, particularly for the liver.

Elder (*Sambucus nigra*): Elder has been described as "a veritable medicine chest" —the flowers, berries, and bark can all be used for different conditions. Elderflower and elderberry wines are two of the most popular country wines, and a traditional way of enjoying the health promoting benefits of elder. Elderflower is used to treat colds and influenza, and because of its healing action on catarrhal inflammation elderflower is also good for hayfever and sinusitis. Elderberries have a similar action to that of the flowers, and are also useful for rheumatism.

Fennel (*Foeniculum vulgare*): During the Medieval Ages fennel—called fenkle—was used to ward off evil spirits. There are many references to fennel in both European herbals and early Chinese medicine. Fennel is primarily

Herbal Lore

According to Greek mythology the beautiful nymph Mentha attracted the attentions of Pluto, whose jealous wife Persephone then trod her viciously into the ground! Pluto then changed her into a wonderful herb.

used as a digestive aid. It relieves gas and colic while stimulating digestion and regulating appetite. A compress, made with an infusion of fennel, over the eyes reduces inflammation of the eyelids. Fennel aids the flow of breast milk but avoid during pregnancy.

Garlic (*Allium sativum*): One of the most useful of all plants in herbal medicine, garlic has an amazing reputation. It is perhaps the most effective antimicrobial plant and it counteracts bacteria, viruses and intestinal parasites. Truly "nature's antibiotic," garlic is used to fight colds and respiratory and alimentary infections. It also lowers blood pressure and cholesterol levels.

Ginger (*Zngiber officinale*): A popular and warming spice, ginger promotes circulation and digestion. Use it as a tea or tincture—or you can make your own ginger beer—to help digestion, tummy upsets, or gas and wind. It is also a common treatment for nausea, morning sickness, and motion sickness. If you have a cold coming on, it will help to promote sweating and detoxify the body, and later,

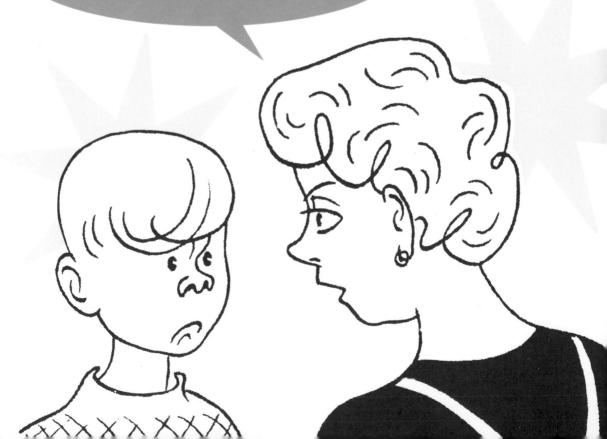

No, darling, garlic does not attract vampires, it scares them away!

if necessary, can help to reduce coughing. Ginger is very good for the stomach and liver.

Lemon Balm (*Melissa officinalis*): The name *Melissa* comes from the Greek word for bee, because bees are much attracted to the scent of the flowers of lemon balm, and produce wonderful honey from the nectar. Paracelsus, a 16th-century German physician, called melissa "the elixir of life." Lemon balm is a carminative herb that relieves spasms in the digestive tract. It relieves anxiety and depression and is a most useful herbal remedy for stress and tension.

Marshmallow (*Althaea officinalis*): This is the herb, not the sickly-sweet soft candy toasted on the end of a stick by children at barbecues! Marshmallow soothes irritated mucous membranes throughout the body, and is particularly used for gastritis and colitis where it soothes the inflamed colon and reduces pain. It also works effectively against bronchitis and irritating coughs, soothing the accompanying sore throat.

Meadowsweet (*Filipendula or Spiraea ulmaria*): This plant is a natural analgesic because it contains "nature's aspirin," a chemical called salicylic acid. This aspirin-like action is effective in

reducing fever and relieving rheumatic pain. Meadowsweet is also one of the best digestive remedies available. It reduces excess acidity, relieving heartburn and gastritis, and helps combat nausea.

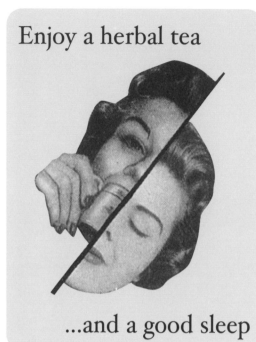

Enjoy a herbal tea

...and a good sleep

nervous tension, and reduces fever and relieves headaches in colds and influenza.

Rose Hips (*Rosa canina*):

Rose hips are freely available from the garden. They provide one of the best natural sources of vitamin C, and help the body to fight off colds and infections. In our grandmother's time rose hip syrup was made regularly, and administered during winter. Rose hip syrup make a good tonic for debility and exhaustion.

Sage (*Salvia officinalis*): Sage is the most effective remedy for treating inflammations of the mouth, throat, and tonsils, also helping with bleeding gums and canker sores (mouth ulcers). Sage also aids treatment of laryngitis, pharyngitis, and tonsillitis. Sage should be avoided during pregnancy.

Senna (*Cassia senna*): Though most herbs have a variety of actions, senna has one that

Nettle (*Urtica dioica*): Despite their bad reputation as prolific weeds that give an unpleasant sting, nettles are a most useful herb. They are one of the best all-round tonics for the body, and contain both iron and vitamin C. Nettles are also astringent and can help relieve nosebleeds. They have a beneficial effect on nervous eczema, possibly owing to the presence of naturally occurring histamine.

Peppermint (*Mentha piperita*): Peppermint is so widely used in products such as tooth-paste, chewing gum, and candy, that its aroma is comforting and familiar. Peppermint is a great remedy for nausea, whether digestive, morning, or travel sickness. It has a tonic effect on the nerves, easing anxiety and

Herbal Lore

The name "salvia" comes from the Latin root word for salvation. Sage earned this name because it was considered so powerful a remedy that it could save people from illness and even death. The Romans called sage, "herba sacra" or sacred herb.

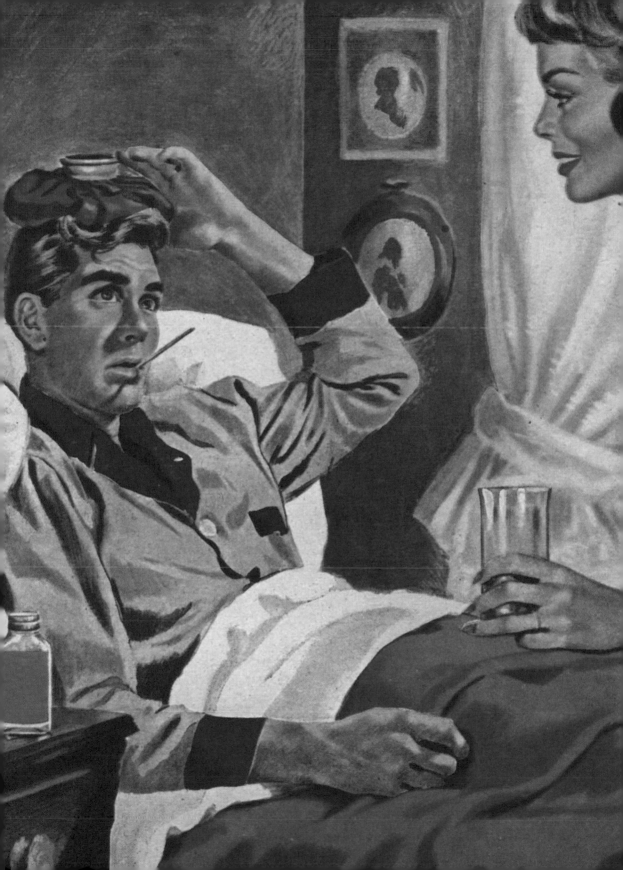

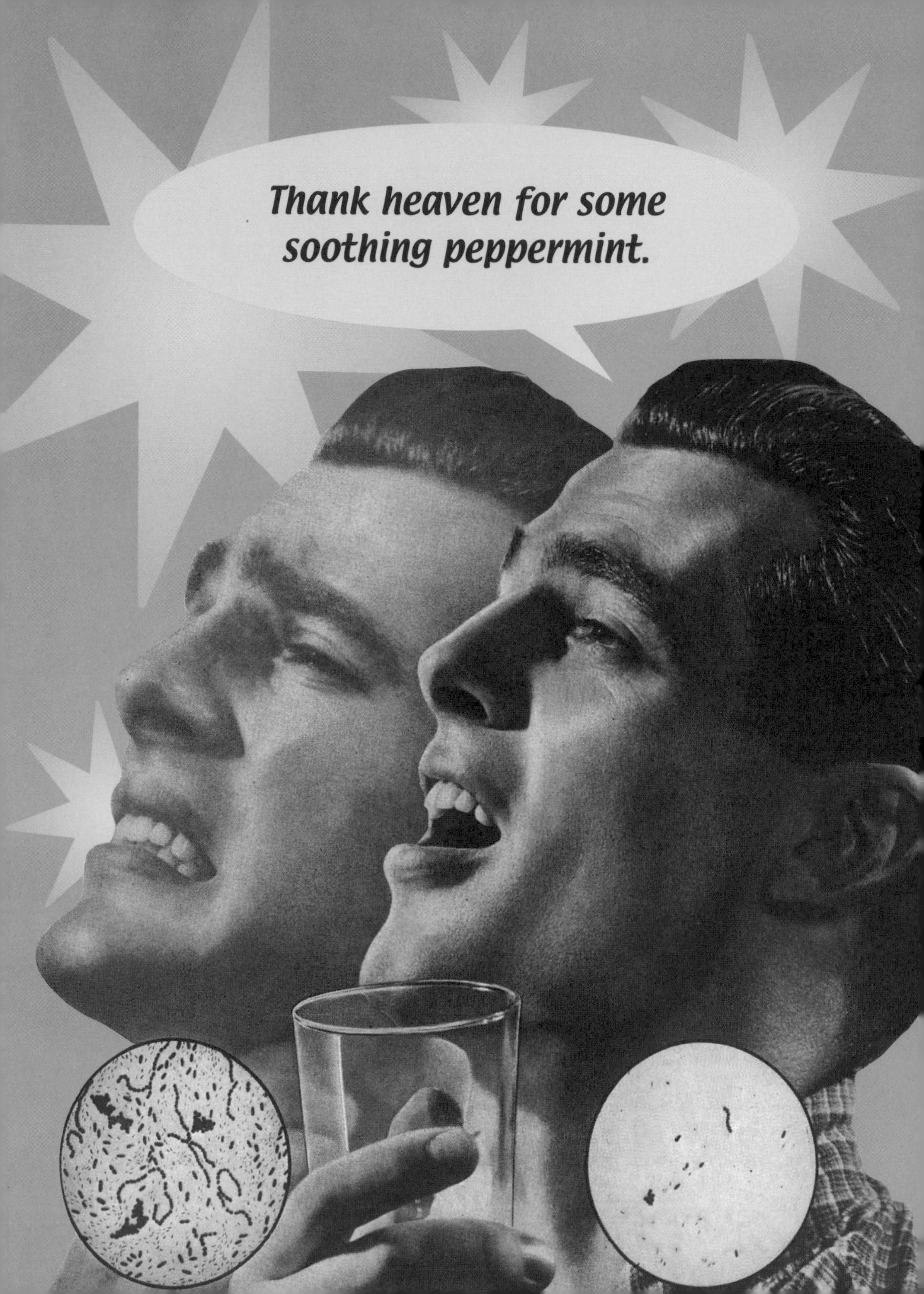
Thank heaven for some soothing peppermint.

Valerian (*Valeriana officinalis*): Valerian has been a highly esteemed herbal remedy since medieval times, and used to go by the name of "all heal." Described in the *British Herbal Pharmacopoeia* as good for "conditions presenting nervous excitability," valerian is an excellent sedative and aid for insomnia. It is also administered for pain relief, especially when the pain is aggravated by tension, and safely combats tension and mild hysteria. Valerian works in many cases by promoting a deep and restful sleep, during which the body heals itself.

predominates, and for which it tends to be used almost exclusively. Senna is the classic treatment for constipation, because it is an excellent laxative. It is the first choice for easing constipation except when this is part of a cycle of Irritable Bowel Syndrome (IBS), when senna might aggravate the symptoms and should be avoided.

Skullcap (*Scutellaria spp.*): This herb is one of the most powerful nervines, or nerve tonics, at our disposal. It has a dual action that is effective in treating stress, exhaustion, depression, and nervous tension. Not only does it induce a relaxed state, it also renews and revivifies the central nervous system. Though this is definitely not to be tried at home, medical herbalists have been known to treat seizures, epilepsy, and hysteria successfully with skullcap.

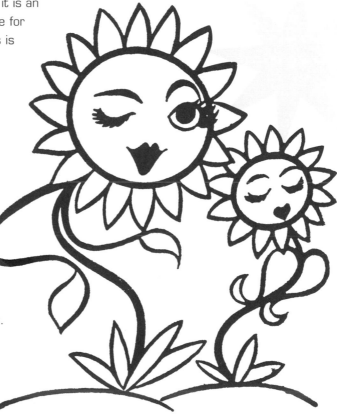

Essential Oils

Essential oils have become popular because their medicinal properties can be easily enjoyed: in the bath, through massage treatment, as additions to lotions and washes, or in the heavenly aroma created when they are heated in burners. You can find them in your local health store, gift shop, or as ingredients of toiletry products in the local store. But what do they do?

Aromatic essences occur naturally in a wide variety of plants throughout the world. When the plant matter is distilled, usually by steam distillation, the resulting vapor provides a essential oil. Essential oils therefore contain the essence of the plant in a form that is highly concentrated and easy to use. The main difference between herbs and essential oils lies in their power and strength; essential oils are many times more powerful than herbs, and are not to be taken internally. They are also used in very low dilutions, typically around 3%, in a base oil, lotion, or cream. When used safely and correctly, however, essential oils have wonderful therapeutic qualities and form an indispensable part of the modern home herbal.

The essence of the plant is what gives it many of its characteristics and has often been described as the plant's personality, or blueprint. With distillation the spirit or soul of the plant is transferred to the essential oil, which therefore contains the precious, vibrant life force and energy of the plant. Thus, essential oils contain the most ethereal and subtle nature of the plants they come from. Consequently, essential oils work on our human higher, subtle levels of mind, emotions, and spirit as well as having a therapeutic physical effect on the body. So the use of essential oils is truly holistic, as the essence of the whole plant is harnessed to heal the whole human mind, body, and spirit.

Some of the most popular healing herbs such as chamomile and peppermint also produce essential oils, so in a few instances an herb is also listed as an essential oil. However, it is important to note that the use and the effect of the herb and the essential oil is quite different. For instance, the most common use of the chamomile herb is to drink an infusion of the dried flowers as a tea, but you would never take essential oil of chamomile internally.

The most appropriate uses of chamomile essential oil are diluted in a base oil for a bath or massage, or in a skin cream or lotion. A hot compress over the abdomen for menstrual cramps or cystitis using chamomile oil is also helpful, and you can drink an infusion of the herb at the same time. Combining the use of the herb and the essential oil in this way increases the effectiveness of each, so long as the proper guidelines for using the herb and the essential oil are observed. The following list incorporates a selection of the most important and commonly used essential oils.

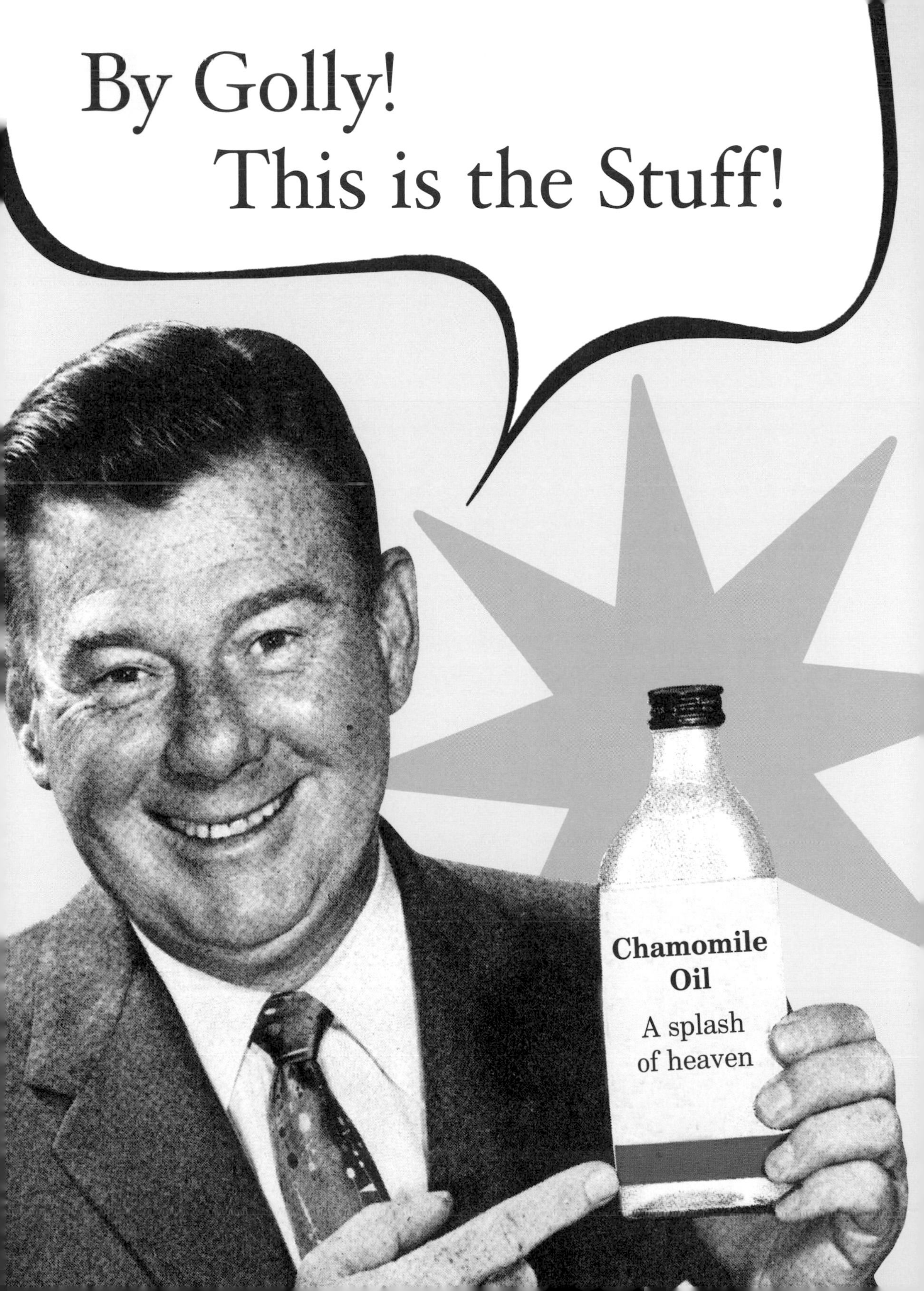
By Golly!
This is the Stuff!
Chamomile
Oil
A splash
of heaven

Wise Woman's Tip

Queen Cleopatra of ancient Egypt used the aphrodisiac power of rose oil to seduce Mark Antony. She is reputed to have sailed down the Nile to meet him with the sails of her ship impregnated with rose essential oil. The wise woman today can use the subtle but powerful scent of rose oil as an aphrodisiac perfume.

Bergamot (*Citrus bergamia*): Though there is an herb called bergamot, the essential oil is derived from a small citrus fruit grown in Italy. Bergamot has three valuable uses: it helps to combat urinary tract infections and cystitis; it gently alleviates anxiety and depression; and bergamot's gently astringent qualities make it effective in skin care.

Headache?

Chamomile Roman (*Anthemis nobilis*) and **Chamomile German (*Matricaria chamomilla*):** Chamomile is soothing, antiallergic, and anti-inflammatory. It is used to treat cystitis, hayfever, eczema, and stomach and menstrual cramps. It is helpful in skin care and in relieving tension and anxiety. Avoid during early pregnancy. It is particularly safe and can be used, if diluted, on children

Eucalyptus (*Eucalyptus globulus*): The piercing smell of eucalyptus is familiar to most people. It is mainly used in steam inhalations to relieve the symptoms of colds, influenza, and sinusitis. Eucalyptus is also an effective insect repellant.

Frankincense (*Boswellia carterii*): Frankincense has the ability to slow down and calm breathing, hence its use in religious ritual to induce a meditative state. It is used to treat respiratory infections and coughs, and helps asthma sufferers by calming them down and slowing their breathing. Frankincense is also valuable in rejuvinating complexions, smoothing wrinkles, and balancing oily skin.

Geranium (*Pelargonium graveolens*):
Geranium is a great balancer of the body's functions, especially the hormones and sebum production. It is therefore much used in skin care and for menstrual problems, including irregular periods and menopausal symptoms. Geranium also stimulates the lymphatic system and is a diuretic, so it is useful in detoxifying and cleansing the body. Avoid during early pregnancy.

Juniper Berry (*Juniperus communis*):
Juniper has a strong detoxifying effect and is a diuretic. It is also a powerful urinary tract disinfectant and useful in the treatment of cystitis, or for preventing the onset of this unpleasant condition. In skin care juniper helps treat acne, and is used commercially in aftershaves. Avoid during pregnancy.

Lavender (*Lavandula vera*): Soothing, balancing, and used for nervous tension and insomnia, lavender is also a most effective treatment for burns. It is used to fight the symptoms of colds, coughs, influenza, sinusitis, and headaches. Lavender is often referred to as a "cure all" because of its many uses. Avoid during early pregnancy.

Marjoram (*Origanum marjorana*): Marjoram is a warming, comforting, sedative oil that works equally effectively on the mind, emotions, and body. It is most commonly used for colds, coughs, and insomnia. One of the most valuable oils to use for massage, marjoram warms the muscles and helps to dispel toxins. When used as a hot compress

Herbal Lore

For thousands of years, lavender has been the most valuable and commonly used of the essential oils. Its name comes from the Latin "lavare," meaning to wash. The Romans used it for cooking, bathing, and scenting the air, it became widely used medicinally in the Middle Ages, and was one of the herbs taken to the New World by the Pilgrims in 1620.

it helps to relieve menstrual cramps. Avoid during pregnancy.

Rose (*Rosa centifolia/damascena*): Roses are associated with love, so it is no surprise to learn that rose has notable aphrodisiac qualities. Rose is quintessentially feminine and has a tonic effect on the uterus, and it is a wonderful addition to skin care preparations. Avoid during early pregnancy.

Rosemary (*Rosmarinus officinalis*):
Rosemary's piercing, stimulating qualities make it helpful in inhalations when there is a cold or sinusitis, and literally "clears the head." Its analgesic properties make it useful in massage for aching muscles, or in a compress for rheumatism and arthritis. It is also good for the digestive system, colitis, and constipation. Avoid during pregnancy.

Oh! My athlete's foot!

Sandalwood (*Santalum album*): Sandalwood is commonly used in incense and as a perfume, but also has a powerful effect on urinary tract infections and cystitis. It is equally impressive as a treatment for dry, irritating coughs and chronic bronchitis. Sandalwood is good in skin care, too, and is a noted aphrodisiac.

Tea tree (*Melaleuca alternifolia*): Originally used by Australian aboriginal peoples, tea tree is a powerful aid against bacteria, fungal infections, and viruses. It is also an immune system stimulant, spurring the body's own defense mechanism into fighting off infections. Tea tree is used to treat vaginal yeast infections, athlete's foot, colds, influenza, sinusitis, acne, and sore throats.

Relieve misery

Herbal Lore

Because rose helps people come to terms with loss, it is particularly good for soothing the emotions and healing a broken heart when a relationship breaks down. For this same reason it is also comforting for those who have suffered a bereavement. Rose is also believed to help women suffering from frigidity.

Bach Flower Remedies

The Bach Flower Remedies were discovered by Dr. Edward Bach, an English physician who had become disenchanted with orthodox medicine. The thirty-eight remedies work on disharmony and negative moods within a person. This extraordinarily subtle method of healing works in a similar way to homeopathy. Both have been proved beyond doubt to be effective, yet neither can offer empirical scientific proof of how they work.

Dr. Bach perceived ill health to have its origins in the mind and emotions. Feelings that are persistently repressed tend to emerge first as mental conflicts, which if untreated go on to manifest as physical illness. A deeply spiritual man, Dr Bach's most cherished beliefs included his famous phrase; "heal thyself" (from Hippocrates), and the central philosophy of treating the person, not the disease. The remedies are all simple to choose and administer, and are selected by observation of mood. They can help to prevent the onset of illness, or if illness has already occurred help heal the person to a point at which the illness dissipates of its own accord. The remedies are so subtle that they rank among the safest of all healing remedies, and incorrect dosage has no ill effects.

The remedies come as a liquid preserved in brandy. Drops usually are added to a glass of water but you can put them in tea, coffee, or soft drinks (unlike most other remedies). You can use more than one remedy at a time, mixing the different remedies in the same glass, but not exceeding the total number of drops recommended. However, taking a larger dose than recommended of any one remedy will not increase its potency.

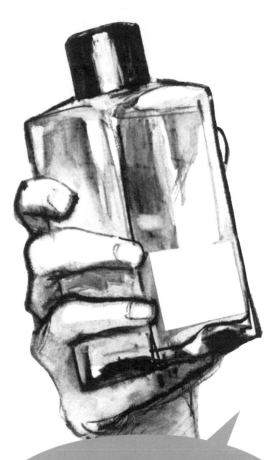

A luxury that actually does you good!

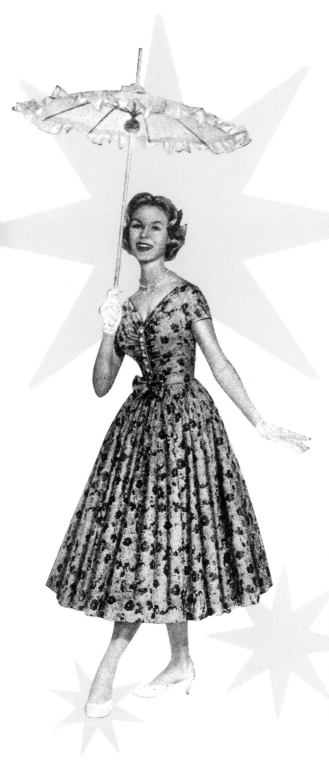

How to use Bach Flower Remedies

To use the Bach Flower Remedies successfully requires no other ability or skill than accurate perception, thoughtfulness, sensitivity, and feeling for the person who is to be treated. The most famous and frequently used of the remedies is Rescue Remedy, a composite of five remedies that work together to combat fear, anguish, and anxiety caused by a sudden crisis, such as accidents, before public speaking and exams, and so forth. As well as the classic remedy to be taken as drops, there is also a rescue cream that can be applied externally to bumps and bruises.

Listed below is a selection of the thirty-eight remedies, that seem especially appropriate for common modern afflictions. The Bach Flower Remedies are easily found in health food stores and homeopathic retail outlets, and a comprehensive range can be found online. It is well worth checking out the other remedies not mentioned here.

Agrimony: For those who try to ignore the dark side of life, or who have problems expressing disappointment and fear. Agrimony also helps those who hide their cares and worries behind a cheerful façade and put on a brave face when confronted with adversity.

Centaury: This is for those who are easily taken advantage of, who are weak willed or who allow others to impose their will upon them. Those who have a tendency to be self-sacrificing or subservient to others are helped by centaury.

Cherry Plum: For those who are plagued by uncontrolled and irrational thoughts. People who fear they may be heading for a nervous breakdown, or feel they may suddenly act violently, are helped by cherry plum.

Crab Apple: For perfectionists, and those obsessed with unrealistic ideals of purity. Known as the "cleanser," it helps those who feel ashamed of themselves. It is also for those who obsess over details, those who "can't see the wood for the trees."

Impatiens: For those—as the name suggests—who are impatient, and quick to irritation with others who do not think or act as quickly as they do. Impatiens helps those who drive themselves and others to the point of exhaustion.

Larch: For those who lack self-confidence and feel inferior to others. Larch helps those who are convinced they cannot do things, so they never even try them, and those who fear failure. It is also for those who are passive and hesitant from lack of self-confidence.

Olive: For those who are drained of energy, in a state of complete exhaustion with both severe physical and mental fatigue, often following a period of extreme exertion or a long illness. Olive helps those who feel that anything more will be "the last straw."

Rock Rose: For those who have been suddenly alarmed, or who are in extreme states of fear, horror, terror, and panic. It is

Herbal Lore

Rosemary was considered sacred by the Romans and used to decorate statues and paintings. During plagues in the Middle Ages it was used to drive away evil spirits. Rosemary stimulates mental clarity and aids thought processes so it is no surprise to hear the old folk saying "Rosemary for remembrance." Today, students in Greece burn it in their homes when they are about to take exams because it has been proved since antiquity to enhance the memory.

for those whose fear is existential or who have irrational fears. Rock rose helps those who have just awoken from a nightmare.

Vervain: For those who are overenthusiastic to the point where they strain their energies and tire themselves out. It is also for those who hold single-minded beliefs and wish to convince others of their principles.

Walnut: For those who are moving on in life. Walnut helps people to adjust to transition and change, during times such as puberty, divorce, moving home, and so forth. It is also for those who have made a firm decision to move on, but are now feeling unsure.

White Chestnut: For those who can't let things go, and are plagued by unwanted thoughts. It helps those who remain preoccupied with a troublesome event, or are still worried long after it happened. Also for those who have obsessive inner mental arguments and dialogues without resolution.

Willow: For those who feel bitter and resentful about the way their lives have turned out. They begrudge their friends and colleagues success and happiness, and even when their own lives do go well they would rather concentrate on the negative aspects than enjoy their good fortune.

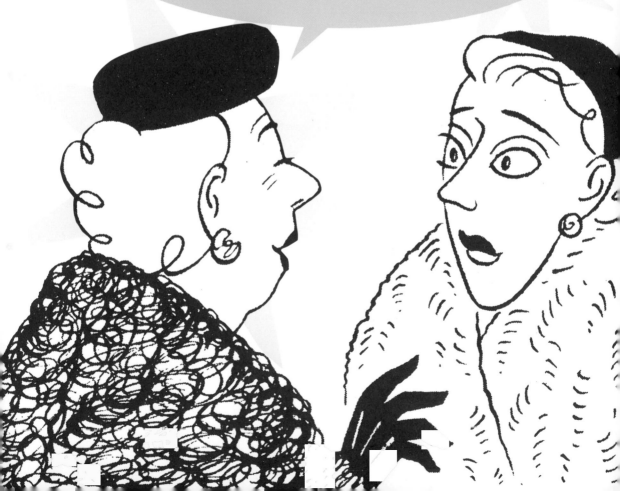

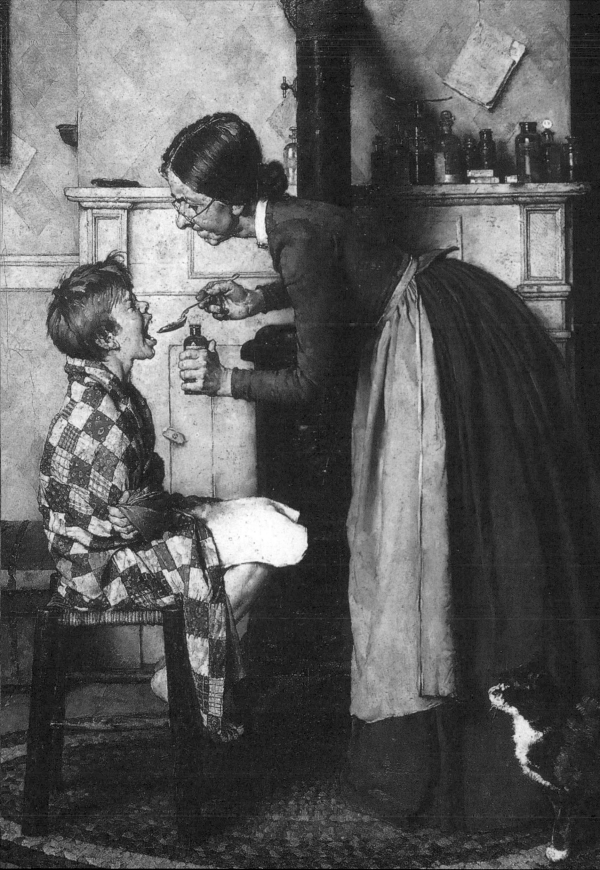

chapter 2

How to Prepare and use Herbal Remedies

Let's Get Started!

Gardeners among you will, no doubt, jump at the chance to grow herbs to create your own herbal remedies. But even if you're not green-fingered there is much joy to be had from making home remedies of infusions, decoctions, tinctures, tonic wines, syrups, and essential oils, using ingredients purchased from your local health store. The more you practice, the easier it will become and the more confident you'll feel. So, let's get started!

Thanks to the proliferation of natural health food shops and herbal suppliers these days, it is easy to obtain a wide variety of herbal preparations. Purchased and used with the greatest of ease, such products give the instant gratification our modern consumer culture expects and demands. Often, in our busy lives, this is all we have time for, and some important remedies need to be bought ready-made in any case, as they are too complex to make at home. Ready-made remedies make valuable, natural additions to the medicine chest and home herbal.

However, the creative art of herbal healing practiced by healers in the past means preparing your own simple herbal remedies. Taking the time to make your own herbal concoctions is deeply rewarding, self-empowering, and a lot of fun. Spending time growing, gathering, or even just purchasing herbs and then preparing them gives you some quiet, thoughtful space and time. This in itself is a healthy counterpart to the hectic and stressful schedule most of us endure from day to day. The herbal remedies you make with your own hands enhance the quality of your life and well-being in wonderful and sometimes unexpected ways.

Knowing how to prepare herbs properly is essential. There are various techniques and methods to use with different herbs, and different parts of the plants, to release their healing qualities the best. The principle of holism discussed in chapter one (see page 13) is also of relevance here. If an herb is prepared incorrectly, not all of its desired healing properties will be present in the resulting remedy. The active properties of an herb exist together in a synergistic, interdependent way involving the whole plant, so the therapeutic ability of the herb lies in its entire being, which is more than the sum of its individual parts.

Infusions

The simplest and most common herbal remedies of all are infusions, and if you know how to brew a pot of tea, you know how to make an infusion. It is an easy way to ingest herbs, some make a refreshing and delicious drink, while others are an acquired taste. It is more convenient to use dried herbs, but fresh herbs can be infused equally well. You need to triple the quantity of fresh herbs to achieve the same strength as if using dried herbs in an infusion.

It is a good idea to keep a china or glass teapot that is used exclusively for herbal teas and infusions, but a clean, scrubbed teapot, well rinsed, will do. It is important that the pot has a lid that fits tightly, to prevent the loss by evaporation of any volatile oils from the herbs. It is best to make fresh infusions each time they are required, because they are full of the life force of the plant and any microorganisms that get in will spoil them quickly. However, if you want to make enough to last for one day, store the infusion in the refrigerator and heat up when required. Wash fresh herbs carefully before use.

How to make infusions

Infusions are created from plant parts such as leaves thin, nonwoody stems, and flowers. These are known as the aerial parts of the plant. Seeds, roots, and bark are too tough and require other methods, (unless they are bruised or crushed before using). Though a single herb, such as chamomile or peppermint, can be used to make an herbal tea, blends can also be made. Using herbs together often creates a more sophisticated and effective remedy that can work on various conditions, and the combination of different tastes can be quite delicious.

NB Herbal infusions, decoctions, and teas are safe, but some need to be taken in moderation. For instance, herbal infusions

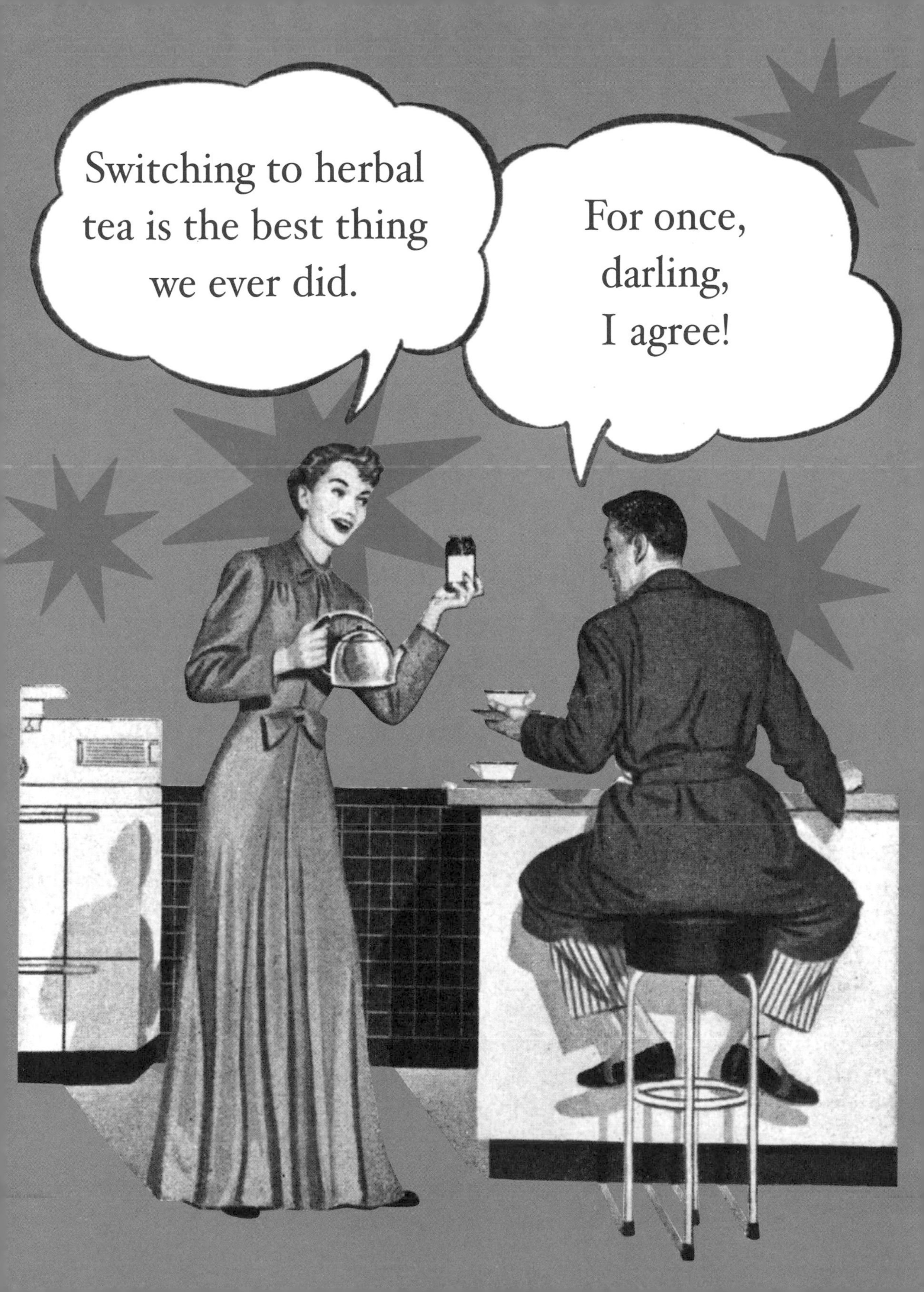
Switching to herbal tea is the best thing we ever did.
For once, darling, I agree!

Wise Woman's Tip

The addition of honey to herbal infusions that have diuretic qualities lessens this effect considerably. For instance, chamomile tea is often drunk before going to bed to promote a deep, restful sleep. However, as chamomile is a diuretic, this can be counterproductive if it makes you wake up to urinate. Simply adding a heaped teaspoon of organic honey to your night-time cup of chamomile tea will allow you to sleep the night through comfortably.

Best drink of the day!

that contain diuretic herbs can overstrain the kidneys if drunk to excess. Sticking to three cups or mugs a day is a good guideline, unless otherwise specified by a qualified herbal practitioner. If you are pregnant, be careful how much you drink—one to two cups daily is best (except with raspberry leaf tea of which three cups a day is acceptable) but avoid all herbal teas in early pregnancy. If you are in doubt or want advice, consult a herbal practitioner.

Before you start making your infusions, you might like to sample some of the ready-made mixed herbal teas available in health food stores, or try experimenting with combinations of some of the following herbs:

■ Flowers of chamomile, elderflower, hibiscus, and lime blossom

■ Leaves of peppermint, spearmint, sage, thyme, lemon balm, and vervain

To prepare an herbal infusion

1) Warm a clean china or glass teapot and put in 1 teaspoon of dried herbs (3 teaspoons of fresh herbs).

2) Pour in 1 cup, (or 1 mug) of boiling water, put on the lid, and leave to infuse for about 10–15 minutes.

3) Strain carefully. The infusion can be sweetened with, for example, organic honey if you like, adding 1–2 teaspoons per cup. Drink hot or cold.

Herbal Lore

Taken as a tea, elderflowers are helpful for hay fever, asthma, sinusitis, colds, and influenza. Elderberries have similar medicinal properties and are useful in rheumatism as well. Elderflower tea can also be beneficial, when an upper respiratory inflammation extends to the ears, causing dulled hearing. Combining elderflowers with anise hyssop and peppermint, makes a pleasant tasting tea enjoyed safely by any age group.

Darling, you add what to your tea..? well I never!

Decoctions

Decoctions are made from roots, seeds, and woody stems. They are usually slightly stronger than infusions, and take longer to make. Because the plant material is hard and tough, the cell walls protecting the plant's active ingredients need more heat and time to break them down and release the healing power of the plant into the water. Decoctions therefore require the herb to be boiled in water. Suitable herbs for decoctions are listed below—you can choose one only or a combination.

Rose Hips, Fennel Seeds, Aniseed, Licorice Root

1) Break, or even grind, the dried herb into small pieces. If using fresh herbs, cut them into small pieces with clean scissors.

2) Take a clean glass or enameled metal (never aluminum) saucepan with a tight-fitting lid. Put in a total of 1 teaspoon of dried herbs, or 3 teaspoons of fresh herbs.

3) Add slightly more than 1 cup or mug of cold water per teaspoon of dried herb to allow for a little evaporation. Put the lid on the saucepan before heating to prevent the loss of volatile oils.

4) Bring to a boil and simmer for 10–15 minutes. Certain herbs take a little longer, and this will be mentioned specifically if such herbs are recommended.

5) Strain the decoction and drink at once, preferably while hot, and sweeten to taste with honey if desired.

Wise Woman's Tip

If you wish to make a mixed herbal tea such as chamomile, vervain, fennel, and licorice, it is best to prepare the herbs separately according to type. You would start by making a decoction of fennel and licorice, then make an infusion of chamomile and vervain. They should then be ready at about the same time, and can be strained into a mug and mixed together, ready to drink.

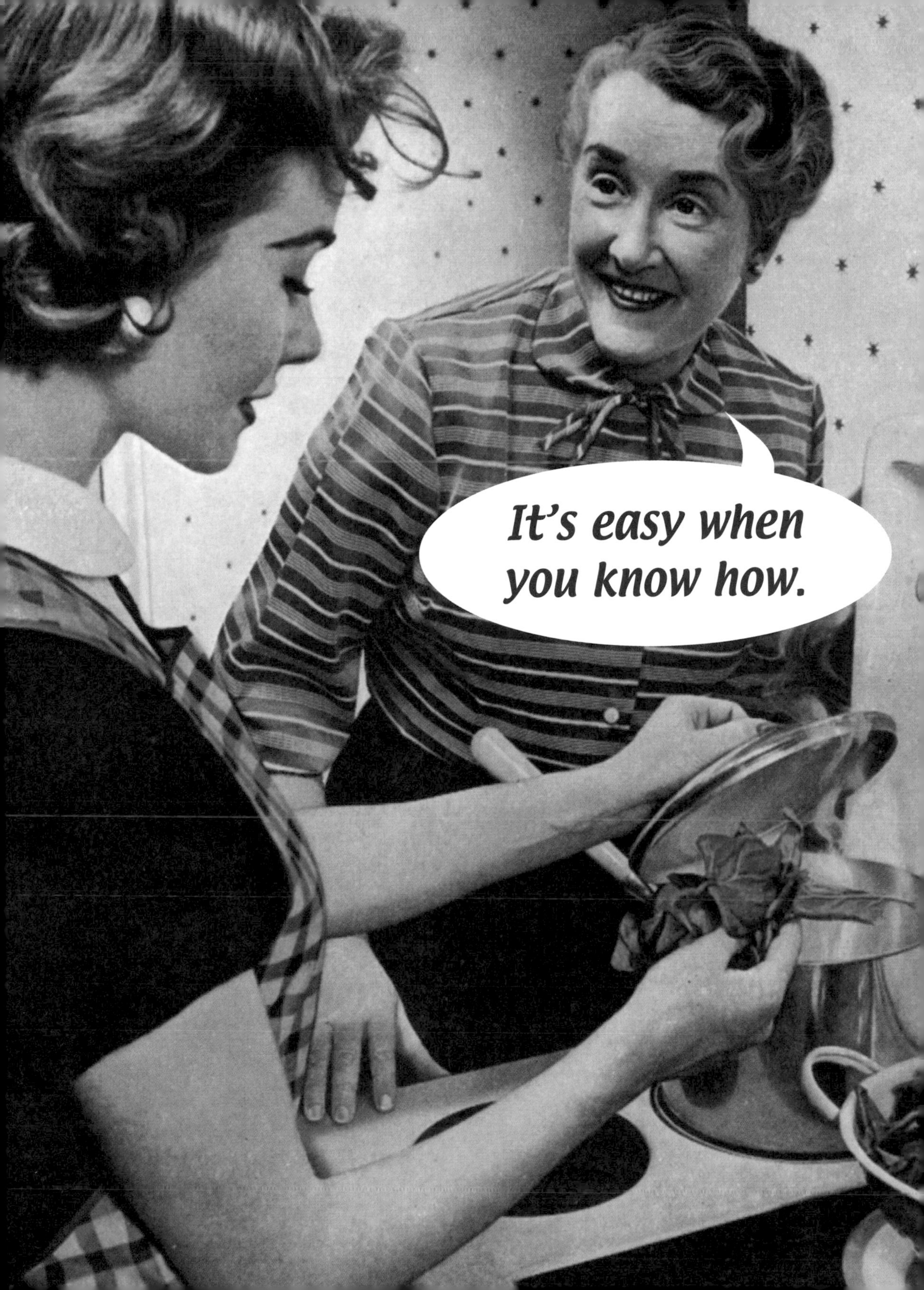
It's easy when you know how.

Tinctures

Tinctures are herbal preparations that incorporate alcohol. The use of alcohol helps to dissolve the active ingredients of the herbs more efficiently than water alone, and, importantly, alcohol acts as a preservative, so that you can make a larger quantity and use it whenever you need to. Tinctures can occasionally be herbal preparations made with vinegar or glycerine, though these are not discussed here, do try some of the recipes that can be found online.

Tinctures are much stronger than infusions or decoctions and only between five and fifteen drops—according to the herb—are taken at any one time. (When specific tinctures are recommended in later chapters, the correct number of drops will be indicated in each case) The drops are mixed into a cup of cold water and then drunk. If hot water is preferred, some of the alcohol will evaporate and cloudiness will appear if the herbs contain constituents that are not soluble in water. This does not impair the tincture, and it should be drunk as normal.

Professionally made tinctures are available in health food stores. These are a lot more specific, and will include their own guidelines on dosage. The alcohol used should be at least 60% proof for preservation purposes. Brandy is used traditionally, but vodka makes a good alternative.

How to prepare tinctures

The instructions given here make simple, general tinctures for home use. As with infusions and decoctions, three doses a day is the guideline, unless otherwise indicated.

1) Take a large sterilized, clean, dark glass jar with a tight-fitting lid.
2) Put in 4oz (120g) of finely chopped or ground dried herbs. If you are using fresh herbs, use 8oz (240g). Dried herbs will produce a stronger tincture in less time than fresh herbs. All parts of the plant may be used to make tinctures: roots, bark, stems, leaves, and flowers.
3) Pour over 1 pint (500ml) of 60% brandy or vodka and screw on the lid tightly. Rum can also be used if you wish to mask a herb

Feelin' Groovy

NETTLE TINCTURE

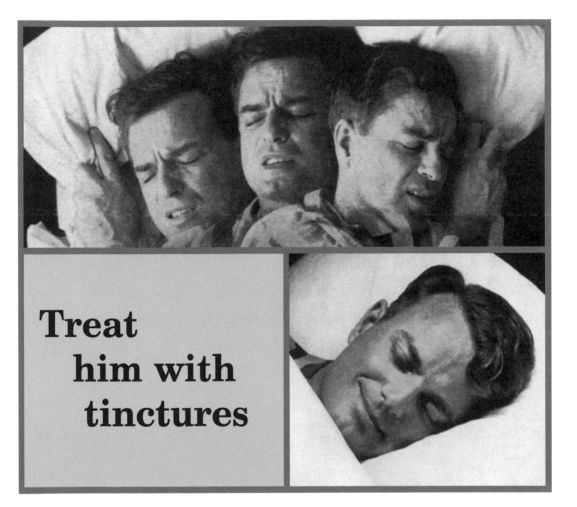

Treat him with tinctures

that has a particularly unpleasant taste.

4) The jar should be kept in a warm place, such as an airing cupboard, for two weeks, and should be shaken vigorously twice a day.

5) After two weeks pour off most of the liquid into a glass jug. Tip the rest into a sterilized clean tea towel suspended over a large bowl. Wring out as much liquid as possible. (If occasionally a stronger tincture is required at the end of two weeks, strain the spent herbs from the alcohol and add new material. Allow this to steep for another two weeks before straining again and storing.)

6) Mix the two liquids thoroughly, then pour the tinctures into one or more glass bottles with dropper caps (this make it much easier!). Remember to label each bottle carefully and clearly with the name of the herbal tincture, together with the date. Store in a cool, dark cupboard and use as required.

Tonic Wines

Traditional country tonic wines provide a more pleasant way to enjoy herbs in alcohol. The long history of these wines is a testimony to their healing powers and delicious taste. The original liqueurs and aperitifs were designed as herbal remedies to aid digestion and stimulate the appetite. Tonic wines fall into two categories: infused wines that it is appropriate to look at here, and fermented wines, recipes for which will be given in Chapter Four, along with other recipes using herbs.

Herbal Lore

Tonic wines were often made in monasteries and the revenue derived from the sale was used to support the monks. Many commercial brands of liqueurs available today are still made to these ancient traditional, and often secret, recipes and contain many different herbs and spices.

How to prepare your own tonic wine

Making your own tonic wine is simple and enjoyable, and a bottle of homemade tonic wine also makes a lovely gift. The following recipe is an adaptation of an old favorite recipe from our grandmothers' time.

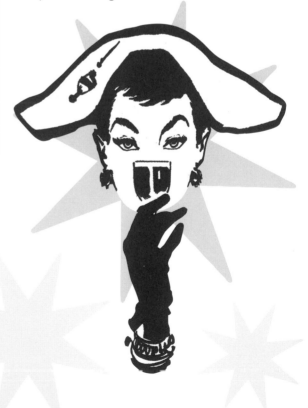

Infused tonic wines are not as strong as tinctures because their alcohol content is lower. This also means that they do not last longer than a few weeks. However, because they are quite delicious and restorative, they tend to be shared with friends and drunk within a few days. A glass or two, when needed, helps to settle the stomach, restores energy levels, and—as all good tonics do—simply makes you feel better. They can even be a hangover cure!

Madeira Tonic Wine

2 bottles of madeira
1 nutmeg, coarsely grated
1 inch of fresh root ginger, peeled and roughly chopped
1 inch of cinnamon stick, broken into small pieces

1 small sprig of fresh rosemary, rinsed
1 small sprig of wormwood, rinsed
15 organic raisins or currants

Take one of the bottles of madeira and pour out one glass. Put all the remaining ingredients into the bottle and replace the cork tightly. Keep the bottle in a cool, dark place—a cellar is ideal—for a couple of weeks. Shake well once after the first week. When the two weeks have passed, strain the infused wine through a clean tea towel into a large bowl, pour in the other bottle of madeira and mix well. Pour into the two bottles and cork tightly. Drink a glass or two as required. You can adapt this recipe according to taste and the ingredients you have on hand.

Syrups

A syrup is basically a thickened version of an infusion or a decoction. Though syrups contain a lot of sugar, which is not very healthy, they are useful to mask the unpleasant taste of some herbs. They also make good throat and cough treatments and children may like them more than traditional remedies.

The simplest way to make a cough mixture or throat syrup is to mix one part of an herbal tincture with three parts of the base syrup, as follows. In a pan (not aluminum) pour in 1 pint (500ml) of water and 2½ lb (1kg) of sugar. Heat gently, stirring until the sugar has dissolved. When it is boiling, take off the heat and allow to cool.

To make a basic honey syrup, boil half a cup of dried herb (whichever you wish to use) in 1 cup of water, then let it steep for 20 minutes. Strain and reboil. Add 3 cups of honey, mix well, and leave to simmer. Pour into a sterilized jar or bottle and seal. To use, add 2 tablespoons to one cup of iced (or hot) water. You can make a soothing syrup from this base by adding a tincture of verbena, hyssop, and wild cherry bark.

Preparing your own cough medicine

For a simple, but effective cough medicine, make an herbal tincture of the herbs listed below and add one part of the tincture to three parts of the syrup. Keep in a dark glass bottle in the refrigerator and take one teaspoon three or four times a day. Use equal parts of: marshmallow leaves, licorice root, aniseed fruit, white horehound leaves and flowers, elderflowers, and thyme leaves.

General Guidelines and Safety Tips

Making your own herbal medicine can be a safe and effective alternative to buying one of the brand-named drugs at the pharmacy—and you know exactly what you are taking! Remember, though, to follow a few guidelines.

If you follow the instructions for taking the various herbal remedies that are detailed in this book, they are quite safe and effective. However, herbal remedies sometimes take longer to have an effect than allopathic medicines, especially with chronic conditions. This is because they work with the body, gently strengthening and stimulating the various body

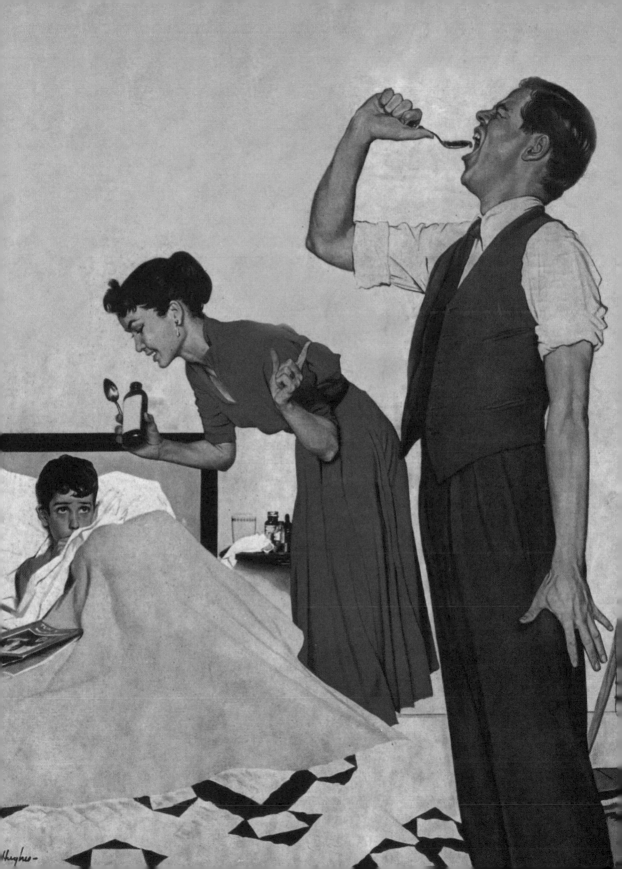

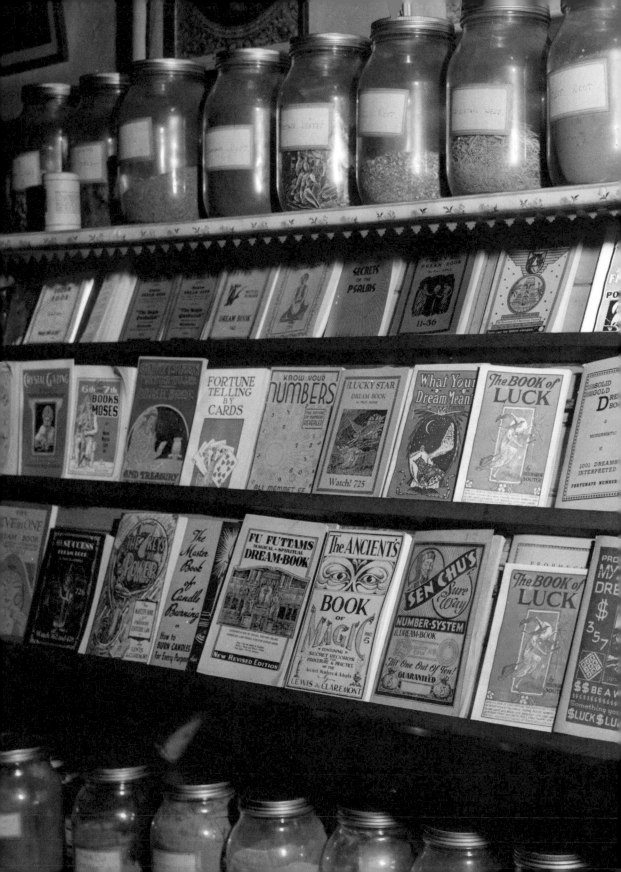

systems, rather than just alleviating or suppressing symptoms. So it is important to resist the temptation to increase the recommended dosage, or to give up because you don't think the remedy is working.

Although you may feel an effect after taking an herbal remedy for a few days, you might not experience the full effects for two weeks, or even a month in some cases. You can try an herbal remedy, and if after a couple of weeks you feel you have experienced all the benefits, it is fine to stop taking it. If you feel it is still helping, continue for a full month. You can gradually reduce the amount taken before stopping altogether, if you like.

It is always a good idea to visit a qualified medical herbalist, who will be able to offer expert advice on all aspects of taking herbal remedies. If you experience any ill effects, stop taking the remedy altogether and see a qualified medical herbalist. If you are taking any medication from your doctor, then you should check with a qualified medical herbalist before taking any of the herbal remedies, except for herbal teas, which are mild and will not affect allopathic drugs. Pregnant women especially need to exercise caution with herbs—even herbal teas—and should always seek expert advice. If you are in doubt, avoid them altogether.

Although the milder herbs are well suited to children, the treatment of children is beyond the scope of this book, so if you wish to give your children any herbal remedies, check with a qualified medical herbalist first. However, the herbal teas of chamomile, vervain, lime flowers, and lemon balm are an exception to the rule and can be given in half the adult dosage to children over six, while teenagers can have the full adult dosage.

How to use Essential Oils

Essential oils are much more highly concentrated than herbs, so developing respect for their potency and an awareness of their suitability before using them is a good idea. Essential oils are simple to use and come conveniently packaged in little glass bottles. This makes them easier to measure out and use than herbal infusions and decoctions. There are several ways to experience the healing power of essential oils, and these are described below.

Aromatic baths

There is something gloriously indulgent about an aromatic bath scented with essential oils, making bathtime luxurious, relaxing, and healing. Many people use oils in their bathwater regularly and enjoy the fragrance and sensations. However, with a little knowledge of essential oils you can take advantage of their healing potential as well.

For morning baths: Bergamot, juniper,

WARNING!
Never take essential oils internally. It is illegal for a fully qualified aromatherapist to advise a client to take essential oils by mouth.

!

petitgrain, and rosemary. Choose one or two. **For evening baths:** Chamomile, frankincense, lavender, marjoram, and sandalwood. Choose one or two.

1) Fill the bathtub as full as you wish with hot water. To stop the oils from evaporating, do not put your essential oils into the bathtub untill you have finished running the water.
2) Mix 6 drops of your chosen essential oils into a teaspoon of base oil, (for example, sweet almond oil or grapeseed oil) and

sprinkle this onto the water. Remember that essential oils don't dissolve in water, so agitate the water before you get in to disperse the oils thoroughly.
3) Step in the bath and enjoy the aromatic bath for 5 minutes or so, breathing deeply and relaxing before starting to wash.

Essential-oil burners

Aromatic herbs have been burned to ward off evil spirits almost since fire was discovered. Gradually our ancestors learned that certain plants made them drowsy, or put them in a trance, and eventually the healing properties of plants was also noticed. The practice of burning rosemary branches to ward off infection was followed in French hospitals right up to the 19th century. Today we can harness the antiseptic powers of rosemary and other essential oils by burning them at home in

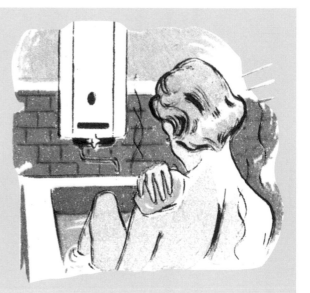

"Mmmm, this is so relaxing!"

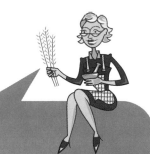

Wise Women's Tip

You can also use essential oils in the shower. Sprinkle up to 6 drops of essential oil, or combination of oils, onto the shower floor just before you get in. The delightful fragrance will mingle with the steam and you will be immersed in an aromatic cloud. Geranium and rosemary are fresh and invigorating for a morning shower, while lavender and chamomile are soothing and relaxing for the evening.

essential-oil burners to ward off airborne infections, colds, and influenza.

Essential-oil burners are made of ceramic or pottery. They have a lower aperture for holding a tea-light candle and an upper bowl to hold water, on top of which is floated between ten and fifteen drops of essential oil. The candle heats the water until the essential oils evaporate with the steam. Inhaling these tiny particles of essential oil vapor has a therapeutic effect. The best way to use a burner is first to fill the bowl three-quarters full of water. You can use hot water if you require an instant effect, but be very careful when dropping in the oils. Otherwise, use cold water. Then light the candle underneath and carefully float the essential oils you have chosen on top of the water.

1) Place the burner in a safe place before lighting the candle—it could be dangerous to move a lighted burner. Not only do you risk spilling the scalding water and oils, but the ceramic burner itself may get too hot to hold comfortably.

2) Make sure the burner is placed somewhere high enough to be out of reach of children and animals. The water will evaporate quickly, even in designs that have quite a large bowl, so it is important to check the burner regularly, and blow the candle out before the bowl burns dry.

Using burners in the sick room

Burners are particularly useful in the sick room because they help the patient to fight off the virus or infection. They also help to protect those nursing or visiting them from catching the illness. Coughs, colds, influenza, sore throats, and sinusitis are all helped by burning essential oils. As well as rosemary mentioned above, lavender, tea tree, frankincense, sandalwood, eucalyptus, thyme, and rosewood are all useful in combating illness. However, you can burn any essential oils simply to enjoy the aroma, and to fragrance a room in a natural and healthy way.

Compresses with essential oils

Hot and cold compresses are a very effective way of using essential oils to reduce inflammation and to relieve pain and swelling. Hot compresses are useful to treat menstrual cramps, cystitis, rheumatic and arthritic pain, localized backache, abscesses, and earaches. Cold compresses are good as first aid for twisted ankles and other sprains, headaches, and any other hot, painful conditions.

Making a compress using essential oils is very simple. Take a bowl of water—either as hot as you can stand to put your hand in, or as cold as possible by placing ice cubes in cold water—and float four or five drops of essential

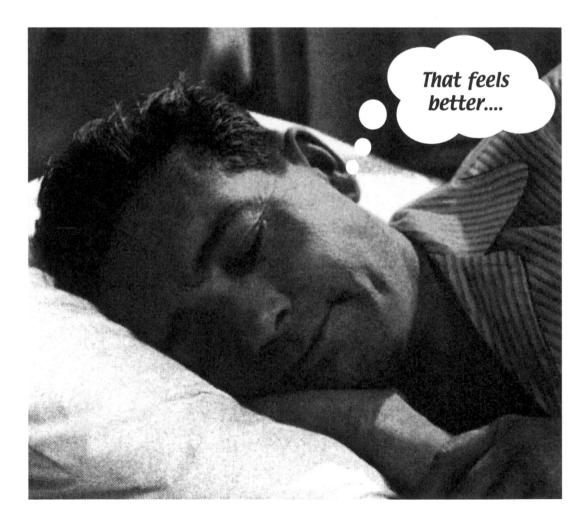

That feels better....

Wise Woman's Tip

You can even use essential oils in a room spray, which creates a more subtle effect than using a burner. Take a new bottle with a spray attachment—or reuse a spray bottle of flowerwater—and fill it with water. Add 10–15 drops of your desired essential oil. Shake well every time before spraying.

oil on the surface. The oil will spread out to make a thin film over the whole surface of the water. Then take a piece of absorbent cloth such as a flannel, handkerchief, or a tea towel and dip it in the water to absorb as much of the floating oil as possible. Wring this out, then apply it to the affected part, replacing it with a new cloth when the compress reaches body temperature.

Alternating hot and cold compresses—with or without essential oils—is a naturopathic technique that stimulates the body's own healing powers. Naturopathy is based on the principle that the body heals itself given the right conditions. A naturopath uses fasting, hydrotherapy, and vitamin and mineral supplements among other methods to promote healing naturally. The following naturopathic technique is particularly effective

with sprains. Start with a few cold compresses as first aid. The next day alternate hot and cold compresses, starting with hot and ending with cold. Lavender is a particularly useful oil for all pains and strains and first choice for headaches, chamomile is good for inflammation, and marjoram is good for aching joints.

Inhalations using essential oils

Steam inhalation by itself is a naturopathic method that fights the viruses that cause colds and sore throats. The addition of essential oils that are antiseptic reinforces the action of the steam, and certain oils stimulate the body to fight off infection. I can remember from my childhood leaning over a basin filled with hot water and Friar's Balsam with a towel over my head, breathing in the soothing fumes. This proprietary remedy, popular in our mothers' generation, is largely composed of benzoin, an essential oil that helps to relieve the symptoms of colds.

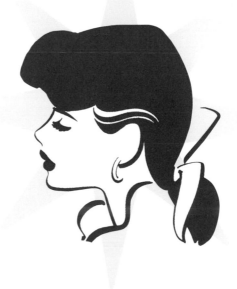

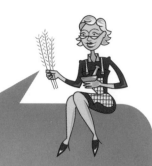

Wise Woman's Tip

If you feel you might be coming down with a cold, or already have one, include eucalyptus or tea tree essential oil in your bathwater. If you have a cough, include sandalwood or frankincense instead.

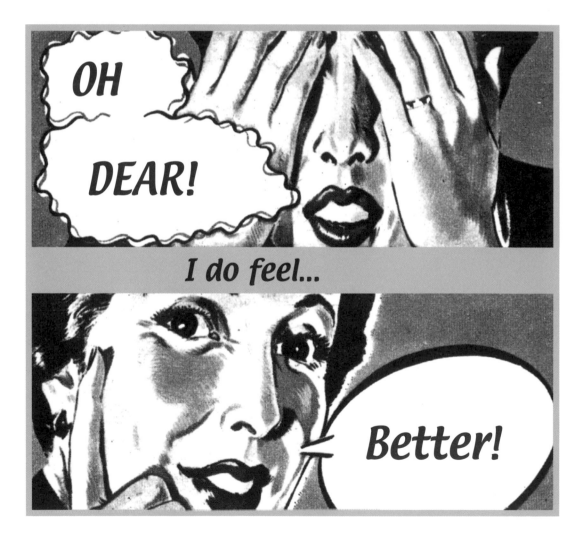

To make a medicinal steam inhalation, take a large bowl, half-fill with boiling water (carefully), and add 3 or 4 drops of an appropriate essential oil. Cover your head and the bowl with a large towel, so that the fumes cannot escape, and inhale deeply for about 5 minutes. As well as benzoin, essential oils of lavender, tea tree, thyme, eucalyptus, and rosewood are all effective in inhalations for treating colds.

How to use Bach Flower Remedies

Bach Flower Remedies should be purchased from a reputable supplier. You can use them in different combinations to create personalized remedies.

The bottles of stock remedy keep well, so you can dilute them as required. Select the remedies you wish to take according to the guidelines suggested in the previous chapter, or those supplied with the remedy. You can combine several remedies, but keep the total number less than six. Take a dark glass bottle with a dropper cap, and fill with natural spring water. Add 2 drops of each chosen remedy to the bottle and shake well. If only using one remedy use 4 drops.

Take 4 drops of this directly onto the tongue without letting the dropper touch the tongue, or in a glass of water, four times a day for as long as required. Hold the liquid in the mouth for a few minutes before swallowing and imagine the remedy as a cleansing light flooding your body with natural healing. The made-up remedy will last about three weeks, but a little brandy can be added to help preservation.

Bach Flower Remedies are completely safe and nontoxic and can be given to children. It can even be given to babies by placing drops in the baby's bottle. Animals and plants also benefit from the flower remedies. For example, Rescue Remedy can be used after traumas such as moving house, accidents, and in the case of plants, being repotted.

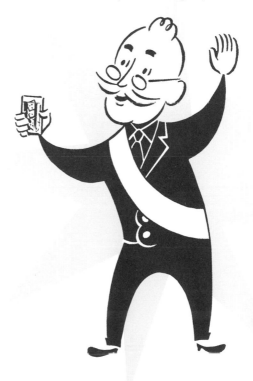

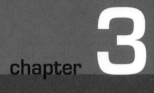

A Modern Home Herbal

Why not Grow and Gather your own Herbs?

Collecting together the ingredients to make your own home herbal can be as simple or as complex as you choose. A modest home herbal might consist entirely of ready-made products, as the range of herbal teas, natural ointments and elixirs now available is comprehensive. However, to follow truly in the footsteps of the wise women healers of the past, it seems appropriate to make an effort to create some of your own natural remedies. A good way to start is to grow a few herbs.

Growing and gathering your own herbs and flowers is a rewarding activity that promotes an understanding and knowledge of herbs and other healing plants. There is something intrinsically satisfying about growing even just a few herbs for use in the kitchen and for drying to keep in your home herbal. The more advanced gardeners can test their skills by creating a formal herb garden, or a traditional herb wheel. You can also find plants growing wild that can be used for treating minor ailments. For example, the active ingredient in the dock plant relieves the stinging sensation of nettle rash. Simply rub the freshly picked leaves over nettle stings until the juicy green sap covers the affected area.

If you have a garden, you can grow fresh dock leaves and other healing plants, but if not, don't worry. Even a humble windowsill can accommodate a few pots of herbs. Some herbs, such as mint, are best grown in pots in any case because their prolific root system can take over a garden. Others such as basil and French tarragon, are delicate and need to be grown either in a greenhouse or in a pot on a sunny windowsill. Below is a selection of valuable healing plants for the home herbal, some of which can also be used in cooking. These can all be grown easily in the garden, and most can be grown in pots and containers on a roof terrace, patio, or windowsill.

Chamomile (*Chamaemelum nobile*): This is best grown as a border plant or aromatic lawn or planted between paving stones, but it is possible to grow chamomile in a large shallow container. Buy young plants. Pick the leaves to use fresh at any time, but gather the flowers to dry when they are fully open in the sun. Use the apple-scented leaves in pot pourri and herbal pillows, and the flowers for herbal infusions and tinctures. The steeped flowers also make a good rinse for blonde hair.

Lemon Balm (*Melissa officinalis*): The lovely, delicate lemon fragrance of the leaves distinguish lemon balm. It is best planted in the border because it grows rather large, though it will do well in a big container. Sow the seeds in spring. Pick the leaves before the plant flowers for using fresh, or for drying.

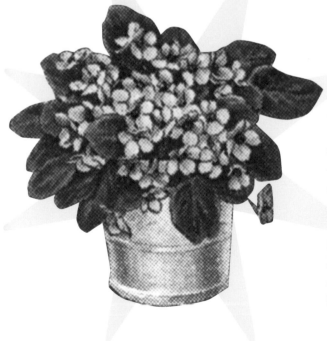

Wise Woman's Tip

Traditional herb gardens were often grown in the shape of a circle, reflecting the concept of holism with an all-inclusive, never-ending design. Sometimes an old cartwheel was used, so the spokes naturally created separate sections, with different herbs growing in each space. A small circular chamomile lawn was often grown in the center.

Lemon balm is very good in herbal infusions, makes a useful tincture, and provides a natural, attractive lemon scent for herbal pillows and pot pourri.

Lime Blossom (*Tilia europaea*): This requires space in the garden. Lime blossom makes one of the most delicious infusions. Large nurseries or garden centers can supply young trees. Gather the blossoms shortly after flowering in midsummer on a sunny day for using fresh or drying. Lime blossom is excellent in infusions and tinctures.

Marjoram (*Origanum vulgare*): This is equally at home in the herb garden or a large container in the sun. Buy young plants. Pick leaves for fresh use at anytime during the

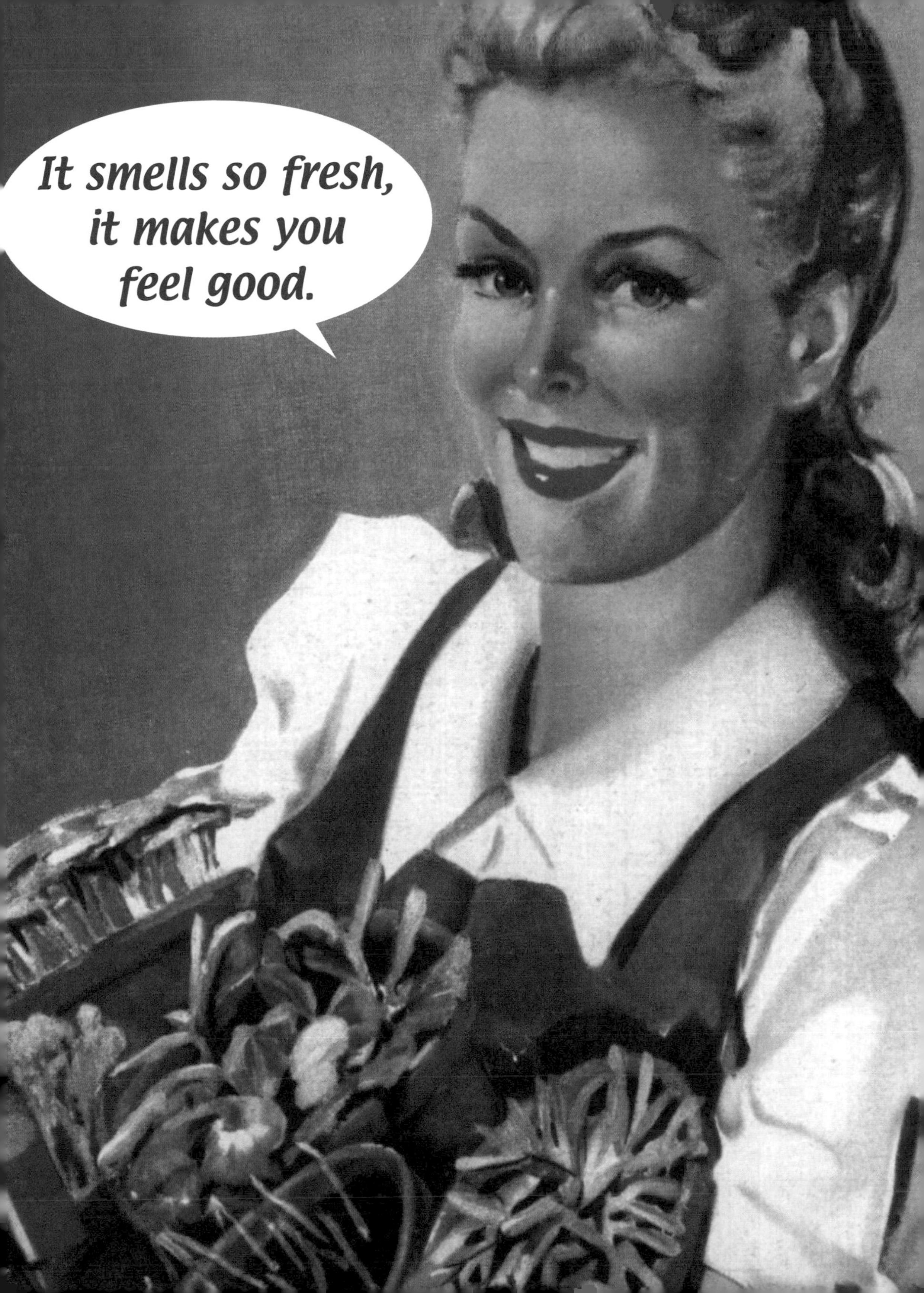
It smells so fresh, it makes you feel good.

Wise Woman's Tip

Choose only the best leaves and flowers for drying, and discard any that are going brown, or have been damaged by insects. Snip off the leaves and flowers carefully with scissors to avoid damaging the plant. Gather your herbs on a day without rain so the leaves and flowers dry quickly and are less likely to go mouldy.

growing season. To dry, gather the leaves before the flowers open. It has many uses in infusions, mouthwashes, gargles, and tinctures, and is commonly used in cooking.

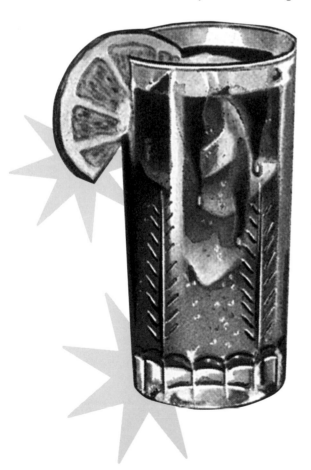

Peppermint (*Mentha piperita*): This grows best in pots, as the roots spread uncontrollably. However, peppermint can be planted in a pot that is sunk in the herb garden if desired. Buy young plants. Fresh leaves can be used at any time, but gather the leaves for drying just before flowering. Peppermint makes an excellent herbal infusion, either alone or in combination, and is also a useful tincture. It adds a sharp, fresh note to herbal pillows and pot pourri and is an indispensable ingredient in certain summer cocktails, such as Kentucky's famous mint julep or the British summertime drink, Pimm's.

Rosemary (*Rosmarinus officinalis*): The powerful scent, needle-shaped leaves, and pale blue flowers make rosemary instantly recognizable. Rosemary is a large border shrub, but it also grows well in a big pot. Buy plants when they are young. Pick the flowering tops at any time during the growing season for using fresh or for drying and storing. You can use it in herbal infusions, tinctures, in everyday cooking, or even as a hair rinse for dark hair.

Sage (*Salvia officinalis*): This is an excellent shrub for the border, but sage will also flourish in a large container. Sow seeds in spring. Pick fresh leaves to use at any time, but gather small young leaves before the flowers open for drying. Use sage in herbal infusions, mouthwashes, gargles, and tinctures. It is also used as an ingredient in various recipes.

Thyme (*thymus vulgaris*): An attractive low-growing small shrub with tiny leaves and pretty, pale lilac flowers, thyme is equally at home in the border or planted in a container. Buy young plants. Pick the leaves at any time to use fresh, but harvest the flowering tops in midsummer for drying. Good in herbal infusions, gargles and tinctures. Culinary thyme is commonly used in cooking.

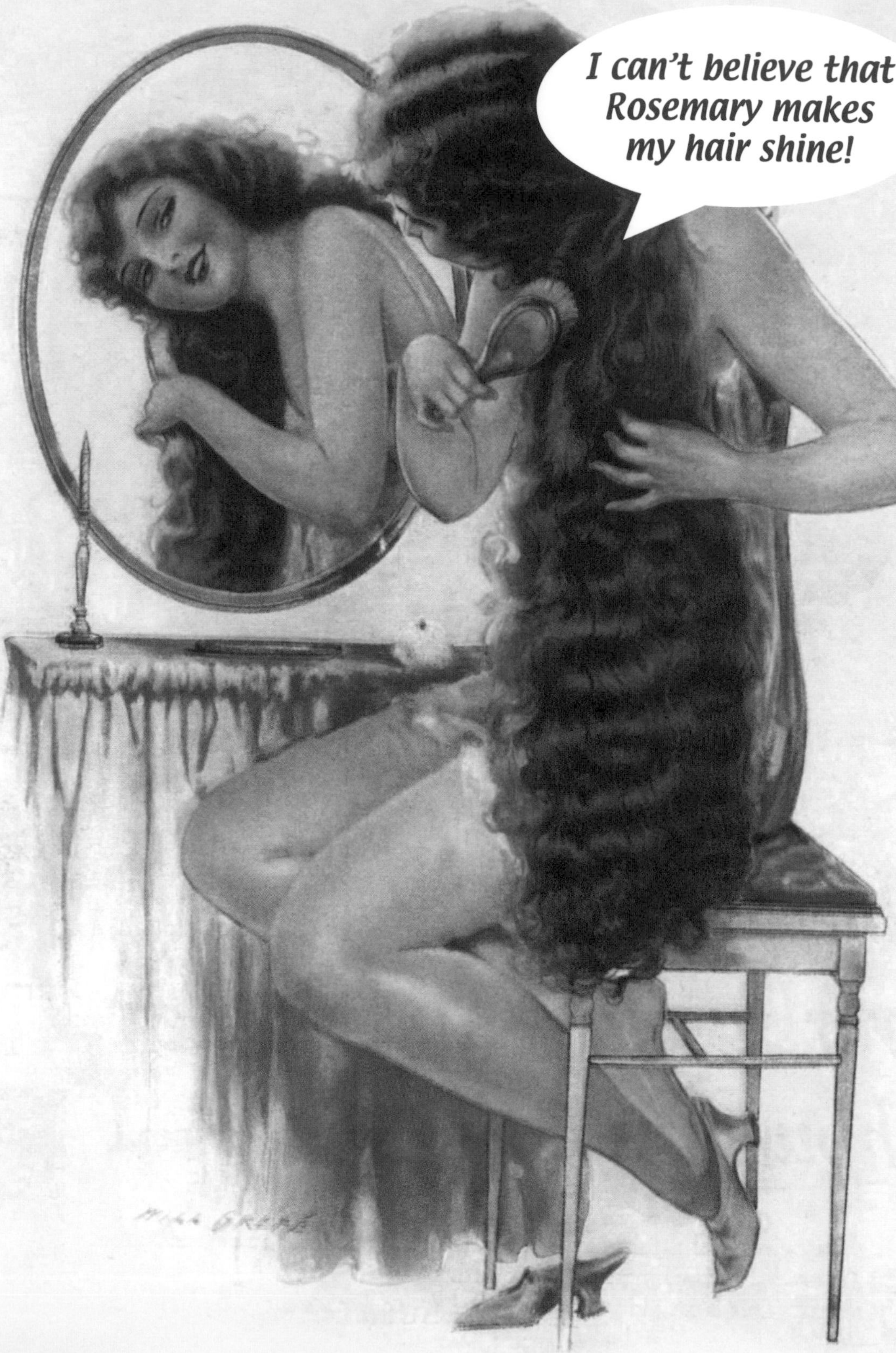
I can't believe that Rosemary makes my hair shine!

Drying and storing herbs

The best way to dry your freshly cut herbs is to spread out the leaves and flowers—leaving some space between them—in single layers. Kitchen wire racks are an ideal base for this job ideal because they allow the air to circulate around the herbs from underneath as well as on top. Do not use artificial heat to dry them more quickly—this dries out the natural oils in the leaves too quickly and spoils the active constituents. You might want to dry a small quantity at a time because it will dry quicker than a large batch.

Herbs come in a variety of sizes and shapes, so the time that it takes for each type to dry will vary. It is definitely best to dry the herbs inside your house to protect them from dust and insects, and also to ensure that they are shaded and will not dry out too quickly, if it is a particularly sunny day. Use separate racks for each herb, and if you are drying several varieties on one day, be careful to label each batch as they are drying, so you don't muddle them up. It is wise to check the herbs regularly, turning the leaves if necessary to ensure the drying process is even.

Once the herbs are fully dried, you should store them immediately. At this point of the process sort through the dried leaves and flowers carefully. Check for any that have discolored badly, or that have dried irregularly. Discard these, and any other leaves or flowers that are not of premium quality. Handle them with care because dry herbs are very fragile and break easily.

The most effective containers for herbs are those that are made of dark glass and have tight-fitting lids. Ceramic or stainless steel containers can also be good. Avoid plastic—any herb that has natural oils might react with plastic. Label each jar with the name of the herb and the date of storing. Keep the jars in a cool, dark place, as part of your home herbal.

Homeopathic Remedies

The great German physician Dr. Samuel Hahnemann (1755–1843) believed that all human beings have the innate capacity to heal themselves, and that the symptoms of a particular illness reflected the individual person's inner struggle to overcome that illness. He concluded that the best medicine would remove the cause of the trouble and stimulate the body's natural healing powers. Shocked by the sometimes barbaric current medical practices of his time, he also sought a form of medicine that would be gentle and safe, yet no less effective. As a result of his quest, and after a number of years of research and experimentation, he established homeopathy.

Homeopathy owes its name to the Greek word *homios*, meaning "like." The basis of homeopathy is summed up in the Latin phrase *similia similibus curentur,* which means "let like be treated with like." Homeopathy is a therapy that treats an illness with a remedy made from a substance that produces symptoms similar to those of the ill person. Homeopaths regard a symptom as the body's reaction to the illness in its attempts to subdue it. Rather than subduing this symptom, then—as allopathic medicine does—homeopaths stimulate this reaction.

Perhaps the most notable difference between the two medical systems is homeopathy's holistic principle of treating the patient, not the disease. Therefore two patients with the same illness may well be treated with entirely different remedies. The homeopath looks at the two patients in terms of their temperament, disposition, and personal characteristics, as well as how each responds to the illness, and prescribes their individual remedies accordingly. There are, however, some remedies that are called "specifics," because these have a specific therapeutic action on a particular ailment and this is common to all people. Among the most common specifics are arnica for bruises, shock, and internal bleeding; and euphrasia as an eyewash for conjunctivitis and other minor eye irritations.

The magic of homeopathy

The magic of homeopathy lies in the use of extremely diluted active ingredients, which are derived from substances that in large doses produce the symptoms of an illness. Some of the remedies are even derived from poisons, which produce symptoms similar to those of certain illnesses. When such poisons are extremely dilute, they act as remedies to treat certain illnesses according to the principle of using like to cure like. In fact, Hahnemann discovered that the more dilute the remedy, the more effective the cure. The most potent remedies are so dilute that no scientific trace of the active ingredient can be found, yet the remedy is still effective. This means that the remedies are completely safe

"Gosh... I think I'd rather be in school"

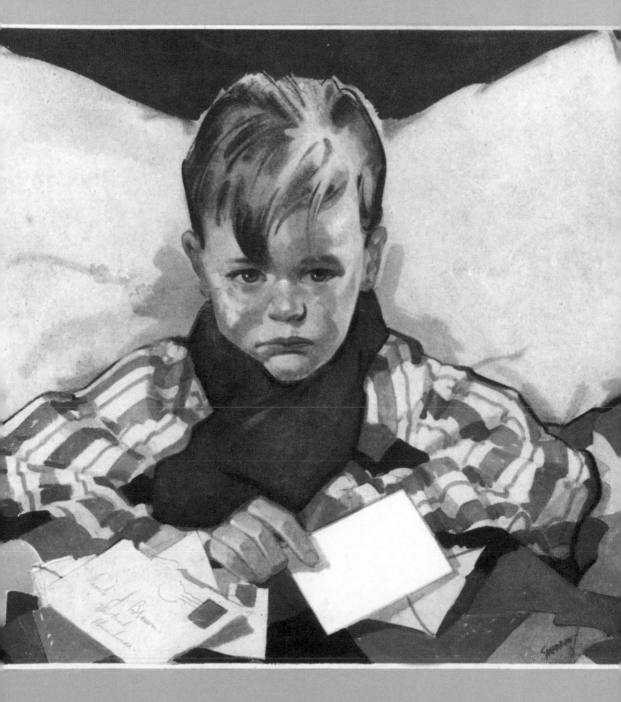

and produce no side effects. They are even safe to give young children.

These remedies are safe and effective to use at home for everyday ailments, and make a valuable addition to the home herbal. Purchase the remedies from a homeopathic pharmacy or a reputable health food retailer. There are several strengths, or potencies; and for self-treatment, use the sixth potency. Take two tablets for adults and one for children three times a day. Dissolve the tablets slowly on the tongue. If the condition is acute, take two tablets every hour for six hours and then revert to the normal dosage. When improvement is noticed reduce the dose and stop after a day or two. Take the remedies between meals, when the mouth is free from coffee, toothpaste, and other strong flavors. If there is no improvement or the condition worsens, consult a homeopathic practitioner or your doctor. Listed below is a selection of commonly used homeopathic remedies for everyday ailments.

Aconite (*Aconitum napellus*): This remedy is useful to prevent the onset of colds after a person has been exposed to cold, damp, and wind. Aconite is also for symptoms that arise suddenly, and for anxiety, bereavement, restlessness, and insomnia.

Arnica (*Arnica montana*): Use arnica after any injury or when physically exhausted after overexertion. Arnica is useful for those who are oversensitive, especially to pain, and for insomnia caused by overtiredness. Take arnica to counteract the effects of shock.

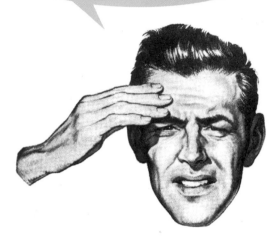

Good for Headaches

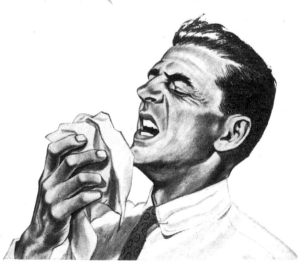

Good for Colds

Belladonna (*Atropa belladonna*):
This remedy is especially
suitable for lively, cheerful
people. Belladonna helps
with throbbing pains,
especially earache, headache,
sinusitis, dry coughs, and the brightly
flushed face these cause. It is also useful
for cystitis and colic in infants.

Calc. Fluor. (*Calcarea fluorica*): This is a
good remedy for colds, especially ones that
are in the head, with thick phlegm and a
mucousy cough. Calc. fluor also helps hot,
itching, varicose veins and hemorrhoids.

Cantharis (*Cantharis vesicatoria*): Use this
remedy for scalds, second-degree burns,
burning pains, and sunburn. Cantharis is
especially helpful for the burning pains of
cystitis and urinary tract infections.

Chamomilla Teething Granules: This is one
of the most effective remedies for fractious
teething children. Because the remedy is so
mild it is completely safe.

Euphrasia (*Euphrasia officinalis*): This comes
as both tablet and liquid. Use the liquid as
an eyewash for any eye irritations; put four
drops in an eyebath with warm water. Use
the tablets as backup for the above eye
treatment. Also use euphrasia when a
streaming cold makes the eyes water and for
symptoms of hayfever. It is interesting to note
that euphrasia is commonly called eyebright,
the name indicating what it is used for.

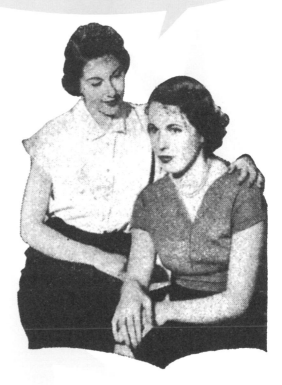

If you're feeling bloated...

Kali. Phos. (*Kalium phosphoricum*): This
remedy is for all symptoms of mental,
emotional, and physical exhaustion, especially
nervous exhaustion. Kali. phos. is also good
for indigestion.

Lycopodium (*Lycopodium clavatum*): This
remedy works especially well for intense,
clever people who are also insecure. Use
Lycopodium for irritability, fear of failure, and

to overcome cravings for sweet food. It is also good for cystitis, menstrual pains, and premenstrual tension.

Nux. vom. (*Nux vomica*): This remedy is well suited to thin, dark people and those who are impatient and quick to irritation. Nux. vom. is good for nerves and oversensitivity, especially nervous indigestion, eating and drinking too much, motion sickness, constipation, hemorrhoids, congestion due to a cold, and premenstrual tension.

Pulsatilla (*Pulsatilla nigricans*): This is especially suited to blond, blue-eyed people with a fair complexion, and those who are affectionate, sentimental, and sensitive. Pulsatilla helps hayfever, all menstrual problems and pains, cystitis, and tinnitus. It is also good for life changes, and when symptoms and moods change rapidly.

Sulfur (*Sulfur*): This remedy is particularly suited to thoughtful, deep people who have a nervous disposition and an independent nature. Sulfur is good for all skin conditions, sweating too much, and body odors; to subdue cravings for rich, spicy foods and candies; to correct energy imbalance; and to normalize bowel movements.

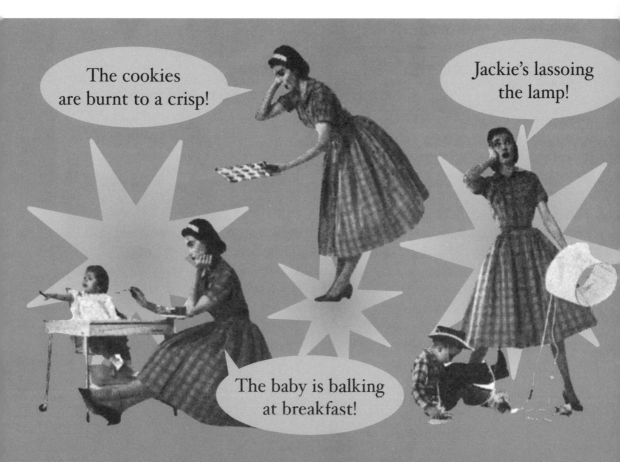

Creating your own Essential Home Herbal

Creating a home herbal is a gradual process of gathering together a collection of natural remedies, and organizing and storing them safely in a suitable place. The kitchen is ideal because most of the herbal treatments require steeping or other preparation, or they are taken with water. Clear out a cupboard that is dark and cool, for storing packets of herb teas, large jars of herbs and bottles, together with a nearby drawer for small bottles of tinctures and tablets, tubes of creams, and ointments. Some people prefer a wooden chest, or cabinet, or even a spacious shelf. The only essential requirement is that the space is dark, dry, and cool, so that the natural products do not deteriorate.

The kitchen provides all the facilities necessary for preparing and taking herbal remedies, but you might like to set aside a teapot, a couple of mugs, and some bowls especially for preparing remedies. There are several basic fresh ingredients commonly found in the kitchen for cooking that can also be used as part of the home herbal. These include: lemons, garlic, cayenne, honey, ginger root, and oats. If you buy these to use in cooking they will also be handy for making natural remedies when required.

Now, what do we have that'll make you better?

Begin with easy-to-prepare herbal teas. For essential oils, start with lavender and tea tree. Include Dr Bach's Rescue Remedy and for homeopathic remedies, include arnica and euphrasia. Listed below are a few other basics for the home herbal, and you can expand on this selection when you feel more confident.

Herbal Teas

There's nothing more soothing than sitting down and having a relaxing herbal tea. And, just knowing how to make your own "special" pick-me-up, will keep you feeling better in itself. Here's some great ideas.

The easiest dry remedies to start collecting are herbal teas. Purchase a few basic herbal teas such as chamomile, peppermint, vervain, rosehip with hibiscus flower, fennel, and nettle. Try to buy organic teas and those free from extra flavors and additives. It is surprising how many "adulterated" herbal teas are on offer these days, where the bulk of the ingredients are synthetic flavorings. Experiment with the different tastes and effects. For instance, see if you like the taste of chamomile tea—with or without honey—and whether or not it helps you to sleep well.

Alongside the herbal teas you can add a few basic dried herbs selected from those already suggested. If in doubt, start with chamomile, lemon balm, and sage. These are the most commonly used herbs and are easy to obtain.

Aloe Vera (*Liliaceae* family)

A traditional "cure-all" folk remedy, this was called the "plant of immortality" by the Egyptians. The juice can be drunk as a general tonic and it helps digestion and mild infections. Aloe has wonderful cosmetic properties (you'll find it in many commercial cosmetics in the local store) and assists the healing of burns. Try buying fresh aloe vera juice, or capsules, skin creams and sun lotions containing aloe.

Calendula ointment

This is an all-purpose healing ointment for minor burns and infected sores; it is very gentle and highly suitable to use on children. For adults you can add lavender essential oil to calendula to help heal burns and scalds, and tea tree essential oil to prevent cuts and grazes from becoming septic. If you decide to add essential oils, use 3 drops per teaspoon of ointment.

Comfrey ointment

This is very good on minor cuts and grazes. Also use comfrey

Wise Woman's Tip

Do not overuse echinacea or other preventive remedies, and avoid taking daily as a matter of course. If remedies are used too often unnecessarily, they will not work as effectively when they are needed.

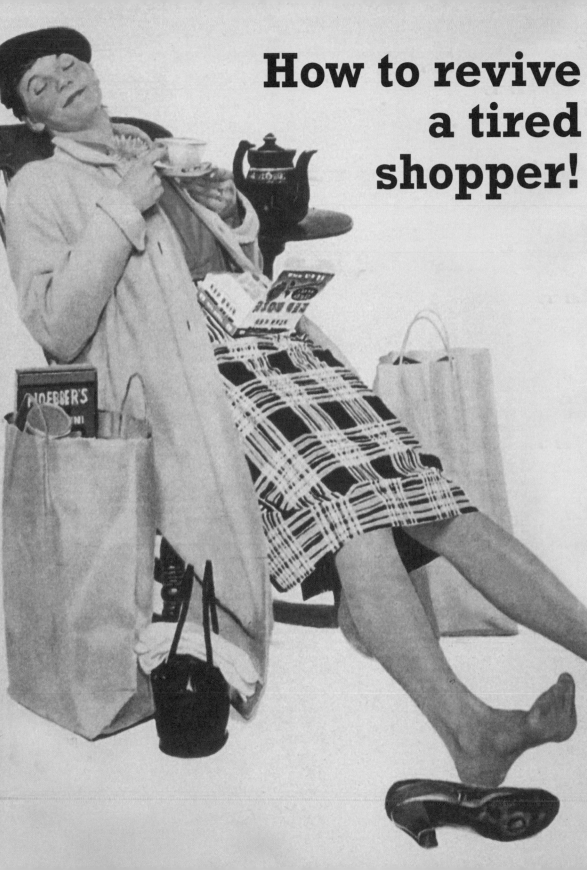

How to revive a tired shopper!

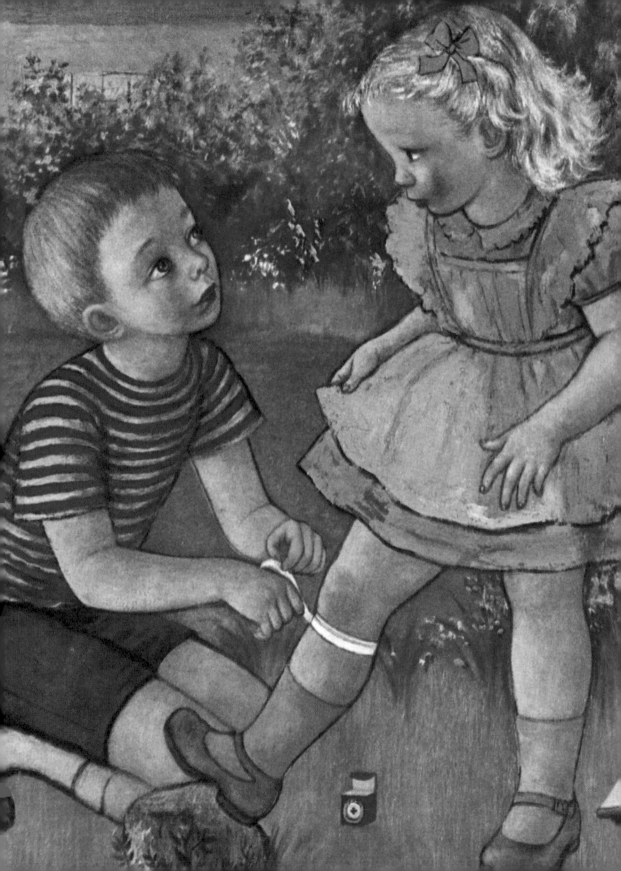

ointment for bruises, sprains, and strains, when it should be applied after using cold compresses as first aid.

Echinacea (*Echinacea angustifolia*)

Echinacea is perhaps the most useful natural immunostimulant. It should be taken at the first sign of a cold, influenza, or other infection, or even when you are feeling susceptible to catching something. It is available in tablets and in tincture form, but the tincture is vastly superior. Take the recommended number of drops according to the instructions on the label.

Evening Primrose Oil (*Oenothera biennis*)

This is not an essential oil, but a valuable supplement containing high levels of gamma linolenic acid. It is available in capsule form and can be taken to treat premenstrual and menstrual problems, eczema, and psoriasis. It is also available as an oil or skin cream, and can be used directly on allergic skin reactions.

Floradix™

This is an excellent all-purpose natural tonic rich in vitamins and minerals, especially useful for people convalescing after an illness. It can be taken at any time to strengthen the body and help to cope with the effects of stress.

Friar's Balsam

This is an inhalant for colds made up almost entirely of benzoin, an essential oil distilled from resin. Though benzoin itself can be used,

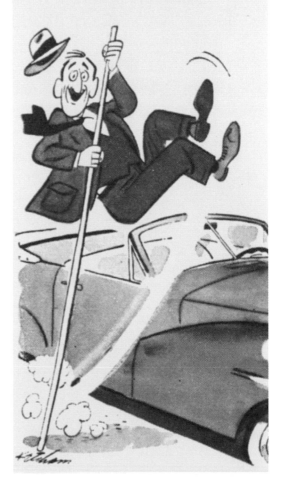

Start the day with a snap!

it becomes thick and sticky quickly and can prove hard to dissolve. Both benzoin and Friar's Balsam leave a yellow stain that is difficult to remove, so keep an old bowl to use for steam inhalations only.

Ginseng (*Panax ginseng*)

This root has been used for centuries to increase vitality and physical performance, and helps to overcome exhaustion and depression. There are two main types available, Korean and Chinese ginseng is generally considered superior. Ginseng is available as a dried root from which a decoction can be made, though tablets and tinctures can also be readily purchased.

Propolis

This is a health-enhancing general tonic that is a by-product of honey and is one of the ingredients of royal jelly. Propolis available in honey and in dried grains, but it is the tincture of propolis that is most valuable. As well as being a natural tonic, tincture of propolis can be diluted in water, adding 4–6 drops to a small cup. Use it as a gargle for sore throats and swallow it.

Royal Jelly

This is also a by-product of honey and is rich in nutrients. Available in capsules or in honey, it can be taken to strengthen the body after illness or as a general tonic.

St. John's Wort (*Hypericum perforatum*)

This is available as an infused oil, tablets, or tincture. The oil is a lovely red color and has a long history of treating wounds, minor burns, and bruises, and is sometimes incorporated into skin care products. The tincture is used as an antidepressant and is reputed to help with Seasonal Affective Disorder (SAD).

Witch Hazel (*Hamamelis virginiana*)

Most commonly used as distilled witch hazel, this is an easy-to-use natural astringent. It can be used as a cold compress on severe bruises, strains, and sprains, and also on minor burns and insect stings. It is often found in hemorrhoid ointments and in varicose vein preparations.

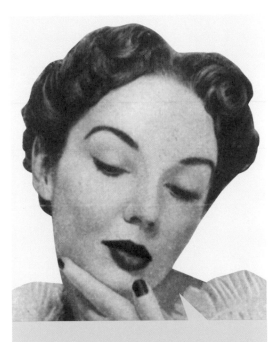

Is your skin parched?

Preventive Health Care

Wouldn't it be great if we never became sick in the first place? That's easier said than done, but while we sometimes don't exercise or eat as healthily as we ought we can help our bodies to head-off sickness before it hits us.

The old saying "prevention is better than cure" applies to many herbal remedies, because they can also be used to prevent the onset of symptoms. Preventive health care is about being really in touch with your body and being able to notice when its natural balance and equilibrium are disturbed in any way. As soon as you sense the first signs of a sore throat, indigestion, or other minor discomfort, take immediate action. By taking an appropriate remedy, you may well prevent the onset of symptoms instead of waiting to see if they will develop into a full-blown cold or infection of some kind.

It is important that you try to have as healthy a lifestyle as possible by eating well, exercising, and generally being kind to your body. In some spiritual traditions the body is regarded as the temple of the mind, and just as you would look after a temple with great respect, so you should look after your body with respect. Remember that it is the only one you have—look after it as well as you can! Luckily, we have access to a multitude of healing plants, and by using them skillfully to maintain our health and well-being we are also respecting, and working with, nature.

A simple lifestyle

Modern society seems increasingly stressful with heavy workloads and commuting, and our cities are often quite toxic with air and water pollution. However, there are some activities that you can undertake that help relieve these pressures, and by doing them regularly you can rediscover the gentle, natural rhythms of life that are more in tune with keeping a healthy mind and body. Simple things such as making time every day to walk in the park or by a river can enrich your life and well-being. Sitting under a tree, listening to the birds, and being immersed in a natural environment help let go of the pressures of the day and allow you time to unwind.

The ancient health-promoting exercise systems of yoga and tai chi are also very beneficial for mind and body. It is easy to find classes in most towns and cities these days, and dedicating an evening a week to discovering the benefits of yoga or tai chi is something most people can manage. The gentle but powerful movements strengthen and tone most of the body systems, and by so doing help to stop imbalances occurring that might lead to ill health. Such forms of exercise also keep the body supple so that even when you are elderly you are able to benefit from doing them. Both yoga and tai chi incorporate a meditative attitude, which itself provides a way to enhance well-being and vitality.

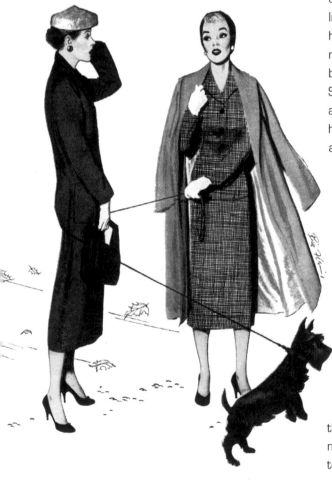

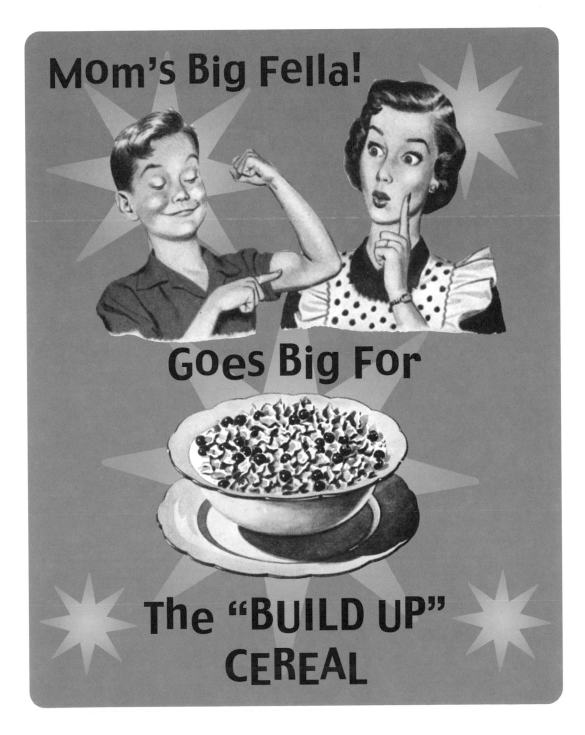

chapter 4

Creating a Healthy Home

Have Fun with Spring Cleaning

The previous chapters have presented ideas and suggestions about herbs and healing plants together with their various preparations, and guidance on how to assemble a home herbal. This chapter takes a step in a different but entirely complementary direction, showing you how to achieve a healthy lifestyle and home environment. You will discover how to use herbs, flowers, and essential oils in a variety of ways to clean and fragrance your home, advice on feng shui, and how to incorporate herbs in cooking to bring their health-giving properties into daily life.

Perhaps the most important part of starting to create a healthy home is looking at what you no longer want to have in your house now that you have embraced the good health magic of healing plants. There is not much point in learning about and using herbs and other natural healing products to enhance your health and well-being, then living an unhealthy life in an unhealthy home. Once again the holistic principle underlying herbal wisdom comes into play, and you can now extend your vision of plant magic to other areas of your life by learning how to use healing plants and complementary practices to enhance your home.

The first thing to do in your quest to create a spacious and balanced atmosphere in the home is to get rid of unnecessary clutter. Many of us have the tendency to hang onto objects that we think may come in useful later. In fact, usually they don't. They just clutter up our lives and gather dust, or lurk in the back of the cupboard. Living with more light and space and fewer material objects can often help to unclutter the mind, and encourage spaciousness into your thoughts. This

enhances your natural creativity, and helps you to appreciate the things that you do have in your home.

There are however, natural objects that bring a special quality to your home. Rock crystals come in many different varieties and

Wise Woman's Tip

Clearing out your home is daunting if you think of it as one task. The best way to approach it is to tackle one small area at a time, such as a drawer or a shelf. If you do this regularly, your home will gradually feel lighter and more spacious, and the pain of parting with your old possessions is minimized.

colors, and are beautiful when placed where the light can catch and reflect their depths. Or you can place a candle in front of them and see how the flickering
flame seems to bring the crystal alive. Polished crystals can be hung up by windows, and a string of small crystals and colored beads can have a wonderful, uplifting effect when the sun suddenly catches them and makes them dance.

Bringing nature into your home in the form of plants and flowers complements their use in healing and cooking. Potted plants—singly or in groups—can dramatically change the atmosphere of a room, and time spent looking after plants can be calming and rewarding. A vase of cut flowers, renewed each week, might seem a luxury, but the effect of the pleasure, freshness, and fragrance of flowers is more precious than the financial outlay.

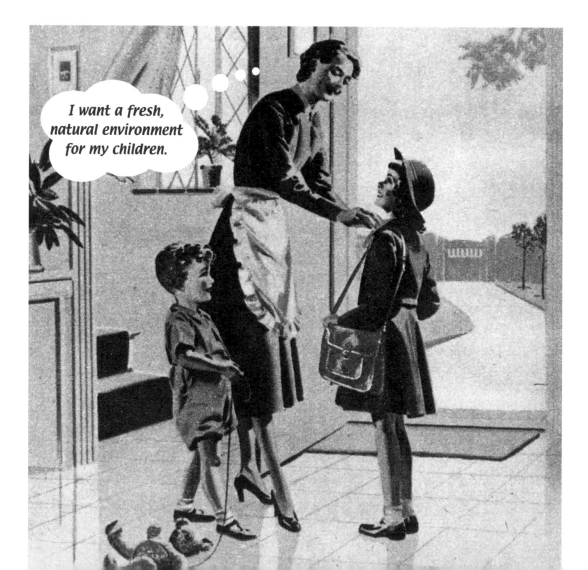

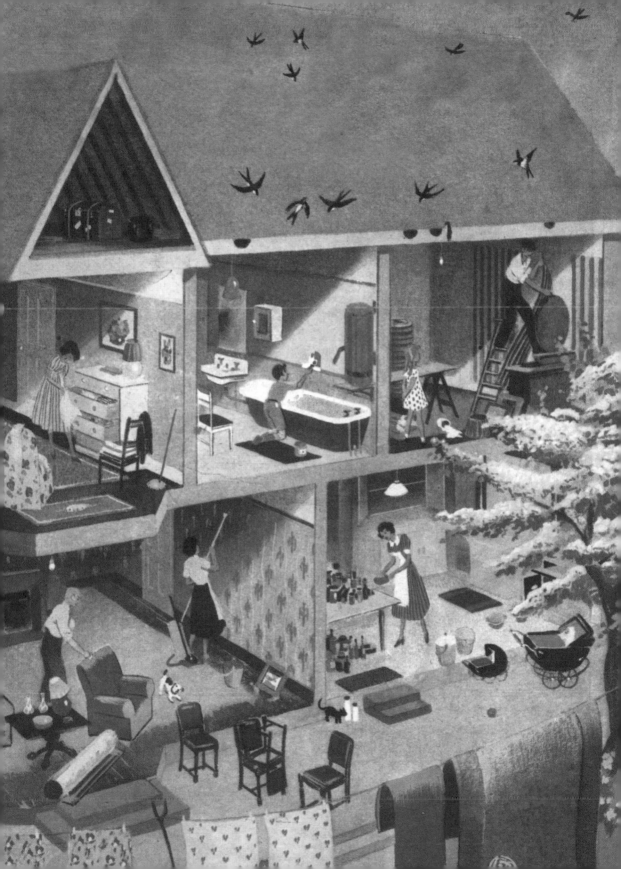

Feng Shui

Feng shui aims to benefit your mental and emotional energies by improving the arrangement of your physical surroundings. Even a basic rearrangement of furniture can have a good influence on the natural chi in your home.

Feng shui is the ancient Chinese art of organizing the space in your home in the best way to allow energy to move freely, which promotes health, happiness, and success. Feng shui means "wind water", and is reputed to have originated some time around 4000 B.C.E. At this time a young Chinese man called Fu Hsi was successful in modifying the banks of the Lo River, which prevented the regular disastrous flooding that often occurred with devastating effects to the region. He subsequently became Emperor as the local area flourished without the flooding, and began to prosper.

Feng shui is a highly sophisticated procedure that involves the feng shui astrology system called Nine Ki and various ancient numerological patterns, together with compass directions to work out how best to organize your home. If you wish to make major changes to the home you are living in, or are about to start the construction of a new home altogether, think about involving an experienced feng shui consultant. The depth of knowledge required to make a substantial difference is considerable.

Alternatively, there are some basic tips that can be drawn from feng shui that are useful for making the most of the natural energies in your home. Feng shui is based on the Chinese belief in the principle of natural energy, the life force known as chi, and the polarized forces of yin and yang. Yin energy is feminine, dark, moist, and passive, while yang energy is masculine, light, dry, and active. At its pinnacle yang energy starts to give way to yin energy, and in the same way yin will start to give way to yang. The symbol that represents yin and yang is a circle, divided in two by a curved line. The yin half is black and the yang half is white, but each contains a small seed of the other, reflecting the ever-changing dynamic of chi.

Chi energy

All things have natural chi, and this is the same energy that we can develop in ourselves by practicing tai chi exercises. The ancient Chinese *I Ching*, or *Book of Changes*, also uses the dynamic interplay of yin and yang as a philosophy of divination. So, how do these chi energies manifest in your home? Chi can be described as the feel and atmosphere of a room, how it is organized, in which direction objects and doors face, and how easily the flow of energy moves between the different rooms in the house. Amending these aspects according to the principles of feng shui can improve the energy of your home. This is the art of feng shui. A number of simple yet effective tips for improving the chi energy in your home are listed on the next pages.

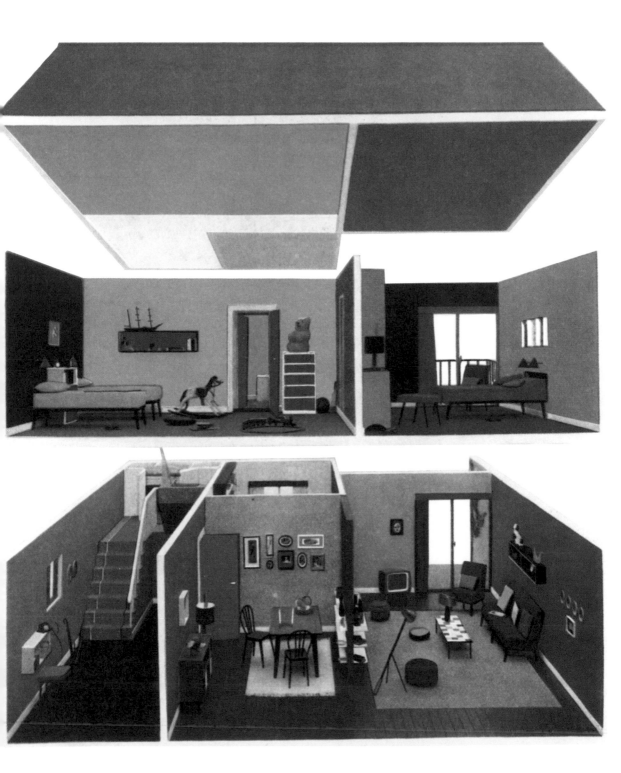

rooms, which corrects the awkward atmosphere and harmonizes the flow of chi in the room.

Lights: These can be used to activate the flow of chi in corners where it can otherwise stagnate, and when light is directed upward it can make the most of the energy in low-ceilinged rooms. Generally speaking, light keeps the chi flowing. Plants work in a similar way, and plants placed in front of corners create a living, vibrant energy. Bushy plants help to slow down chi and can be useful in corridors and near doors.

Mirrors: Never hang a mirror directly in front of your bed because it is important not to reflect back at yourself the chi emanated while you sleep—emanating chi while asleep is the body's way of cleansing and recharging itself. More positively, mirrors can be strategically hung to conduct the flow of chi throughout the house beneficially. For instance, mirrors hung on either side of a long corridor will move the energy from side to side and slow it down, preventing a rushed feeling permeating the area. Mirrors can also be positioned to create the illusion of space in irregularly shaped

Compass direction: The direction a room faces will also have an effect on the flow of chi. Listed below are some simple feng shui guidelines based on which compass direction a room faces.

■ **North** is associated with sleep, sex, meditation, and solitary creativity. Good uses for a north-facing room are a bedroom, an artist's studio, or a meditation room. Unless you want to live a quiet, independent life, your front door should not face north because this can bring feelings of loneliness. The color associated with north-facing rooms is off-white, so this is a good color to predominate in such rooms. A north-facing bed (with the head pointing toward the north) is suited to mature people who are not lonely and who desire quiet, peaceful sleep. It might also help to revive flagging sexual energy.

■ **Northeast** has a sharp, piercing energy, and a shiny, sharp, competitive atmosphere. This is the least favorable direction for a front door. Northeast is associated with playing and physical exercise, so a northeast-facing room would be a good choice for a child's playroom, or an adult's exercise room. The associated color is brilliant white, so shiny gloss paint would be appropriate. A northeast-facing bed is considered inauspicious. Candles add fire and warmth to a room and are particularly recommended for rooms facing northeast.

■ **East** is associated with ambition, strong motivation, and putting dreams and ideas into practice, so the energy is active and focused. A front door facing east is especially suited to young, active, ambitious people. Rooms that are east-facing make good kitchens, offices,

and practical hobby rooms, and an east-facing bedroom is helpful if you want to become busier, or build up a new career. The color associated with East is bright green, like the vibrancy and vitality of a new leaf. An east-facing bed, once again, suits young, active, ambitious people.

■ **Southeast** also has an active energy, but this is persistent and enduring rather than aggressive and ambitious, and suggests an orderly, harmonious energy. A front door facing southeast helps you to develop your life harmoniously and enhances communication. Suitable uses for rooms in this direction are a kitchen or an office, while a bedroom here will gently foster development. The associated color is a dark, mature green, like a fully developed leaf. A southeast-facing bed is auspicious for communication, creativity, and harmonious progression in your work.

■ **South** has a fiery, passionate, and brilliant chi energy, and when this flows well throughout the home it brings fame and social

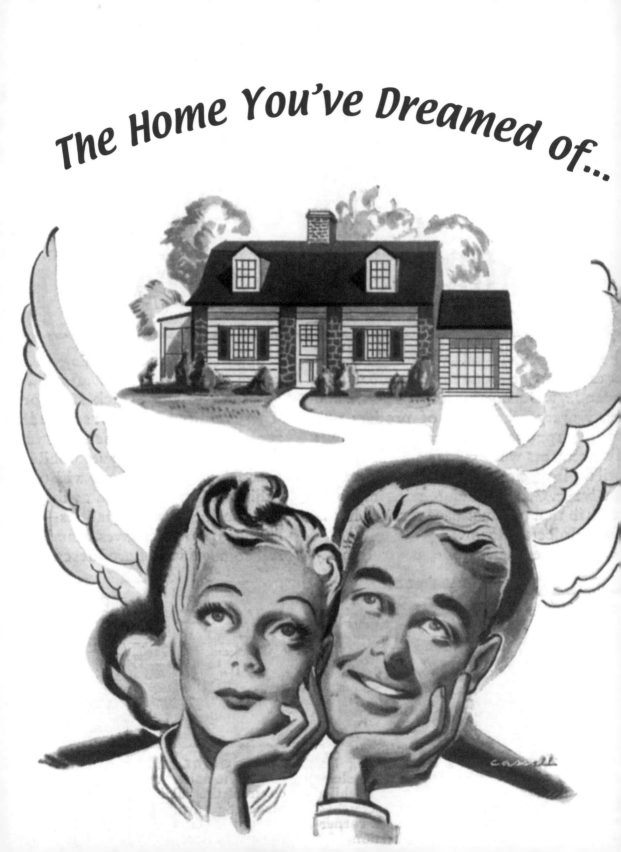

The Home You've Dreamed of...

popularity. A south-facing front door denotes an active social life and favors intellectual creativity, though the fiery energy can sometimes boil over into arguments. Rooms with this aspect are ideal for entertaining and parties, though a study or bedroom might work well for a young, active person. Purple is the associated color. A south-facing bed does not promote restful sleep, but it might suit young, deep-thinking personalities.

■ **Southwest** is associated with a cautious, methodical progression toward harmony, and a slow, steady energy. A front door facing southwest is inauspicious for good health, but rooms with this aspect suit family activities, so any kind of family room is well suited to this direction. Black is the associated color, especially the nourishing, fertilizing color of black earth. A southwest-facing bed is inauspicious, especially for health.

■ **West** is associated with harvest, fulfillment, romance, and money. A front door to the west encourages a settled flow of chi throughout the house. West-facing rooms are ideal for entertainment, such as in a dining room or sitting room, and for relaxing in front of a sunset. A bedroom in this direction might lead to a preoccupation with pleasure at the expense of getting things done. Red is the color of the west, like a beautiful fiery sunset. A west-facing bed leads toward increased contentment, sexual pleasure, and romance, though it may be detrimental for motivation.

■ **Northwest** is the direction of leadership, forward thinking, and orderliness, and the chi energy has dignity, authority, and respect. A front door with this aspect indicates that the occupants can easily cultivate dignity and trust. Northwest-facing rooms make ideal offices, libraries, and studies, while a bedroom here would suit older parents. The associated color is silvery-white, which might be compared to the hair color of wise old sages. A northwest-facing bed suits those who are in positions of authority, natural leaders, and parents, but also for mature people winding down in life.

Wise Woman's Tip

Crystals can be used to improve the energy in your home. Hang them from a beam or window sash to help get rid of bad energies. They can also be used in hallways to slow down or activate chi. Crystals are ideal for improving the energy in a gloomy room or dark corners, as they will attract more light and energy.

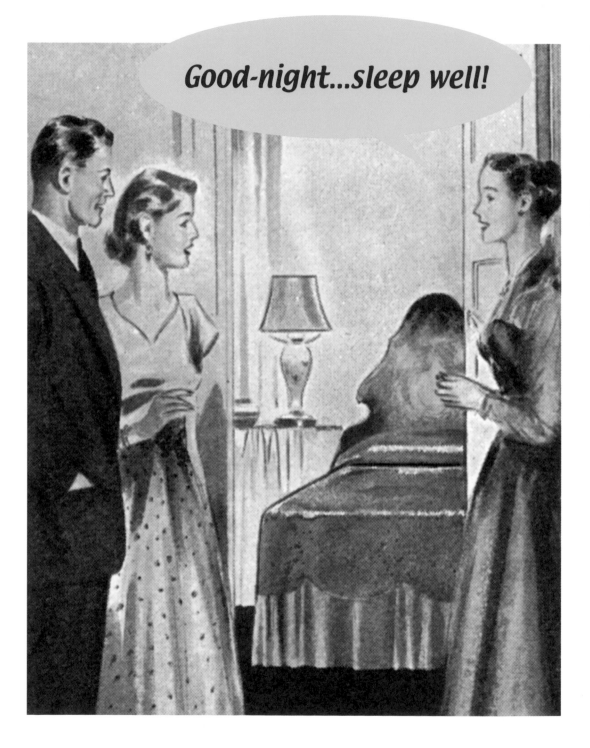

Using Essential Oils in Cleaning Products

Harsh cleaning products with fiercely chemical aromas don't have to be the norm. The addition of essential oils not only improves the smell of your home— they can aid the cleaning process too. From polishing wood to cleaning crockery, many essential oils have a useful function—you just need to know what to do.

Commercial cleansing products are often laden with unpleasant synthetic fragrances, which in extreme cases can cause or aggravate an allergic reaction. Such synthetic chemicals are best avoided as much as possible. Good alternatives are the ranges of natural cleaning products made from biodegradable ingredients, which are not destructive to the environment as well as being gentle to you and your home. However, some of these products go to the other extreme and are unperfumed altogether, which can leave an indefinable bland smell after cleaning. Although this is not actually unpleasant, it can be improved upon safely, naturally, and quite delightfully with the addition of essential oils to natural cleaners.

Certain essential oils are historically associated with cleaning, notably lavender. Lavender has been used to clean wounds, in bathing, and for washing linen for thousands of years. Geranium has powerful insect-repellant and deodorant qualities. All the lemon-scented oils also work as insect repellants and were traditionally used in cleaning products. Unfortunately, these days the sickly lemon scent in many commercial cleaners is synthetic and definitely not as pleasant as real lemon, citronella, bergamot, and lemongrass. Cedarwood and sandalwood essential oils also repel insects.

Personal preference plays an important role in which essential oils you choose to fragrance your cleaning products, so if you don't like the smell of a particular oil—even if it is recommended—don't use it! There is a wide range of essential oils to choose from, and deciding which ones you like is part of the fun of making your cleaning products smell the way you want them to. However, it is important that the dishwashing liquid, floor cleaner, and so forth are free from synthetic fragrances, otherwise you could create something that smells quite awful, and you would still be subject to the adverse influence of synthetic chemicals.

How to perfume cleaners

There are numerous cleaning products that you can perfume. These include: dishwashing liquid, liquid clothes detergent, fabric softener, floor cleaner, all-purpose surface cleaner, and toilet cleaner. One way to mix the essential oils in thoroughly is to keep an old bottle of the product, and then half-fill it from a new bottle. When you add the essential oils you can shake the bottle thoroughly to ensure that the oils are thoroughly mixed in. Alternatively, you can pour the cleaner into a large jug or bowl and

stir the oils in with a spoon or stick, before carefully pouring the perfumed cleaner back into the bottle.

You can use a 0.5 % dilution—or even less if you prefer a subtle scent or you tend to use a lot of cleaner. The dilution can be worked out by using an approximate multiple of tablespoons (15ml). For each 2 tablespoons (30ml) add 2 drops of essential oil. So, for example, a 1 pint (500ml) bottle of cleaner would need about 33 drops of essential oil, or less according to preference. It is very important that the essential oils are thoroughly mixed in, to avoid too much essential oil being used at any one time. For most cleaning fluids you can use whatever essential oils take your fancy. Here are some suggestions:

Dishwashing liquid: Lemon (this is recommended because it is relatively harmless if a faint residual fragrance is left on the dishes, though you should always rinse them well!).

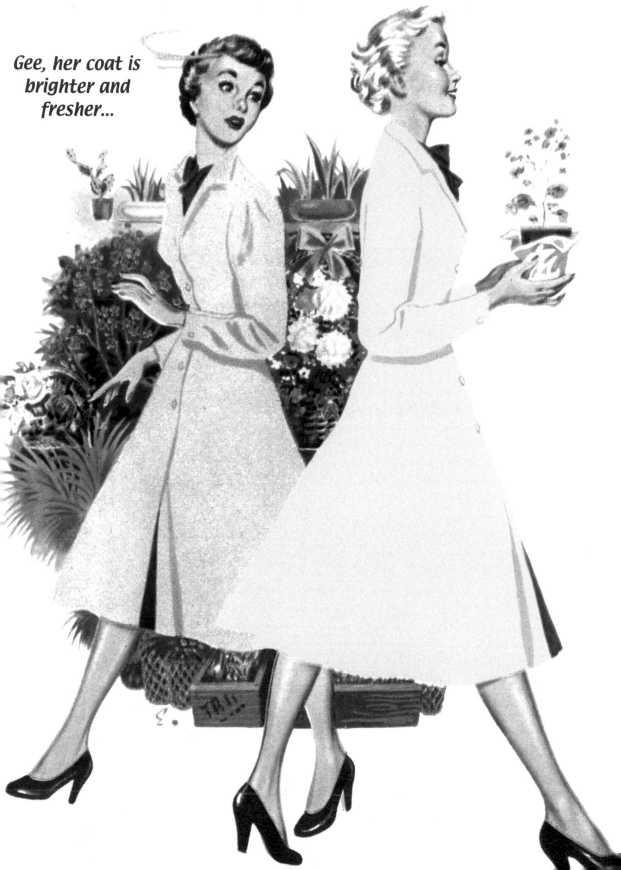

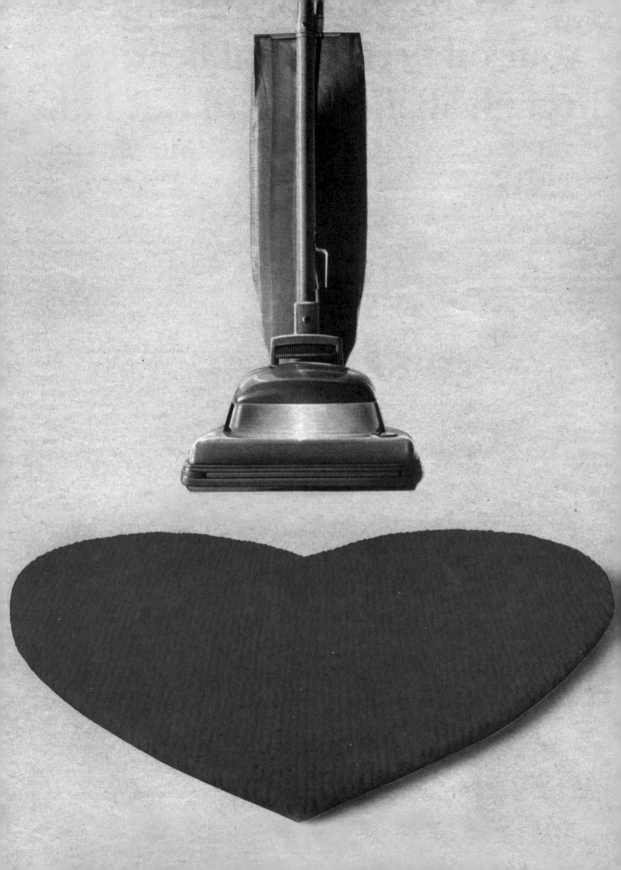

Floor Cleaner: Pine and eucalyptus, or pine and cedarwood, or lemon and juniper.

Fabric Conditioner: Geranium and chamomile, or ylang ylang and rosewood, or sandalwood and lavender.

Toilet Cleaner: Pine and lemon, or juniper and cedarwood, or lavender and thyme.

Liquid Laundry Detergent: Lavender and geranium, or bergamot and palmarosa, or lemon and ylang ylang.

If you would rather not mix the essential oils directly into the various cleaning fluids (especially if you're still at the experimental stage), there are other ways to use them. These methods are also good because they mean that you can choose different oils each time you clean. For example, you can add 3 drops of essential oil to fabric conditioner in the washing-machine dispenser just before you use the machine. You can add 4 drops of essential oil into the bucket of water containing floor cleaner, just before washing the floor. You might even put 3 drops onto a tea towel and put this in the tumble dryer just before drying a load.

How do aromas help?

The essential oils you add to cleaning products don't just smell nice—they can help your mood and have practical benefits. If you need waking up or calming down, the scents you choose can make a difference:

Rosemary and basil—both of these essential oils are stimulants and can help to wake you up or brighten your mood.

Chamomile and lavender—these aromas are relaxing and would be good to use in the home during the evening.

Cedarwood and sandalwood—are both insect repellants so might be a helpful essential oil to have in the home during the summer.

All essential oils are naturally ocurring antiseptics, so they have a good practical use in cleaning the home.

A few pieces of advice to bear in mind:
■ Be careful in the handling of cleaning products and try to choose environmentally-friendly, or natural, products that are not already heavily perfumed. Keep them out of the reach of children.

■ Never get essential oils in the eye. If you do, rinse the eye out and consult a medical practitioner immediately.

■ Avoid bringing undiluted essential oils in direct contact with skin, as an allergic reaction may occur. If you have sensitive skin and you're using essential oils in washing up liquid or clothes detergent, you should start off by using one or two drops only. If there is no adverse reaction you can increase the number of drops gradually.

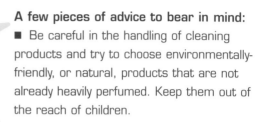

Wise Woman's Tip

When cleaning carpets with a vacuum cleaner, put 4–6 drops of your chosen essential oil onto a cotton ball and place this in the dustbag. The fragranced ball will freshen and perfume the room while you are cleaning.

You are What you Eat

Many people make the mistake of equating healthy eating with bland food. But a little knowledge about herbs and their culinary application soon proves that healthy eating can provide some of the most stimulating tastes available. Don't be frightened of cooking with herbs—they are versatile, readily available in stores or your garden, and, most importantly, delicious.

The old saying "you are what you eat" is as relevant today as it has always been. A healthy, nutritious diet promotes well-being and longevity, and can help to ward off many minor ailments and even more serious diseases.

Though there is no guarantee that eating a healthy balanced, nutritious diet will absolutely prevent the onset of disease, by giving your body the best chance of good health by eating well, you will be doing the best you can.

Modern culture has brought us prepackaged convenience food, and instant-gratification fast foods, which are usually full of saturated fat, salt, and sugar, and, most damagingly, chemical additives. These are toxic for the body. Moreover, when you consider that the whole food chain has become contaminated by all sorts of chemicals, the scenario looks much bleaker. Seeds are coated with chemicals to promote rapid growth and repel insects, the crops are sprayed, the animals that eat the crops are regularly injected with antibiotics, and the meat often has preservatives added. So what can you do to eat a healthy diet?

The step is to consume foods that are as close as possible to their natural state (when they still contain naturally occurring vitamins and minerals), and there is less chance of their being contaminated. Thus, you should eat lots of fresh fruit and vegetables, and as many of these as possible should be eaten uncooked. If you buy only organic foodstuffs wherever possible then you should eliminate many chemical additives. Whole-grain foods, such as brown rice and whole-wheat bread,

are good for you because they are high in minerals and fiber and help prevent constipation.

Try being vegetarian

Most Western adults eat too much protein. Reducing or eliminating meat from your diet is one of the ways to lessen protein intake.

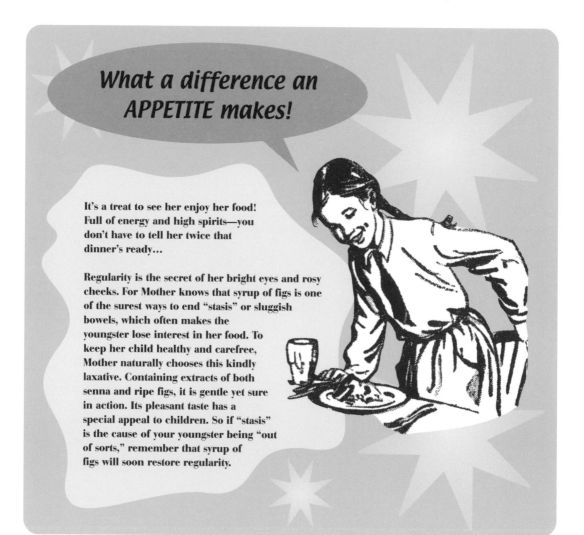

What a difference an APPETITE makes!

It's a treat to see her enjoy her food! Full of energy and high spirits—you don't have to tell her twice that dinner's ready...

Regularity is the secret of her bright eyes and rosy cheeks. For Mother knows that syrup of figs is one of the surest ways to end "stasis" or sluggish bowels, which often makes the youngster lose interest in her food. To keep her child healthy and carefree, Mother naturally chooses this kindly laxative. Containing extracts of both senna and ripe figs, it is gentle yet sure in action. Its pleasant taste has a special appeal to children. So if "stasis" is the cause of your youngster being "out of sorts," remember that syrup of figs will soon restore regularity.

Eating less meat also reduces your intake of animal fats, which several scientific studies have proven to contribute to high blood pressure and coronary disease. There are alternative, healthy ways of getting the necessary proteins required for good health without eating meat such as nuts, soy products, and legumes, while free-range or organic fish is generally less toxic and often healthier than meat. If, however, giving up meat completely seems too drastic, then try to eat smaller amounts and make sure that it is lean, free-range organic meat. Better still, eat chicken and turkey (again, organic or free range is best).

There are other unhealthy foods you also need to eliminate or restrict. These include refined flour, found in cakes and cookies, sugar, salt, caffeine, and those chemical additives listed as e-numbers in the list of ingredients on food packaging. Most of us could benefit from eating less fat, and the fats we do eat should be vegetable, such as extra virgin olive oil for cooking and to dress salads, and organic sunflower spread instead of butter. Of course, such a strictly healthy diet may prove difficult to stick to at all times, but it serves as a good basis for healthy living.

Giving up meat and prepackaged foods laced with artificial flavorings could lead to bland-tasting meals, but the addition of herbs can help. Not only are herbs good for you, they also add natural flavor to many dishes. Most culinary herbs stimulate and aid digestion, and have been used successfully in cooking for many generations. Eating garlic regularly helps to fight off colds and infections, and to lower high blood pressure and cholesterol levels.

Listed below are a few common culinary herbs that you can grow on your windowsill or in the garden. Why not aim to develop the habit of using them in your daily cooking?

Basil (*Ocimum basilicum*): This is one of the best culinary herbs for a sunny windowsill, where plants will grow prolifically. Sow seeds in late spring. Basil is used extensively in pasta dishes and salads, and is the main ingredient of pesto. Snip leaves to protect the plant, and then simply tear or pound the leaves with a mortar and pestle as required.

Chervil (*Anthriscus cerefolium*): The subtle flavor of chervil leaves is reminiscent of parsley and anise. Seeds can be sown

Aromatic Stewed Peppers

Take 2 red peppers, 2 yellow or orange peppers, and 1 green pepper.
Remove the seeds, then chop the peppers coarsely into 1-inch pieces. In
a heavy-bottomed frying pan, sauté 2 or 3 finely chopped garlic cloves in
2 tablespoons of extra virgin olive oil on a low heat. Add the chopped peppers
after 2 minutes, stir well, and cover the pan. Stew gently for 15 minutes,
stirring occasionally to prevent sticking. Add a little water if necessary. Take
a handful of tarragon, or other herb, strip the leaves off the stalks and chop
them finely. Add to the peppers, stir well and leave for another 5 minutes.
Add freshly ground black pepper and a tiny amount of salt if desired. Serve as
a main dish accompanied by rice or pasta, or as a side dish, or starter. It is
delicious served either hot or cold.

throughout spring and into summer. Chervil grows quickly and easily runs to seed, so use the leaves from young plants to achieve the best results. Use finely chopped chervil in egg, vegetable, and fish dishes, also in salads, soups, and sauces.

Chives (*Allium schoenoprasum*): These can be grown in a large pot, or as a low, edging plant for garden borders. Sow seeds in spring. Chives are a quick-growing culinary herb with a mild onion flavor, and the long, narrow leaves can be cut freely and chopped finely to bring flavor to salads (great in potato salad!), dips, and soups. Chives are also very good mixed into soft cheese, and the edible flowers can be used decoratively in salads.

Dill (*Anethum graveolens*): This herb has distinctive blue-green feathery leaves and an aromatic, tangy flavor. Sow seeds through spring into early summer, and use the leaves from young plants before they run to seed. Dill is a traditional ingredient of potato salad and fish dishes, and is also good in soups and sauces. The seeds, as well as the leaves occasionally, are an indispensable ingredient of homemade pickles.

French Tarragon (*Artemisia dracunculus*): This is a delicate plant and is best grown in a pot that is left sitting on a sunny windowsill, or in the greenhouse. Buy young plants because the only seeds available to buy are often **Russian Tarragon (*artemisia**

dracunculoides) which has a vastly inferior flavor. Tarragon is traditionally used in "fines herbes," sauce béarnaise, and tartar sauce, and large sprigs are used to infuse white wine vinegar. Tarragon also imparts a lovely flavor to vegetable and chicken dishes.

Parsley (*Petroselinum crispum*):
Perhaps the most commonly used herb, parsley grows easily in a pot. Because of its high vitamin C content parsley is a healthy, useful herb that can be cut freely and chopped finely into many dishes. Sow seeds from late spring into early summer.

Opposite is a simple, delicious, and healthy recipe in which you can substitute the tarragon for basil, chervil, or flat leaf parsley. Or you could be creative and use a selection of different herbs! The more you experiment with herbs, the easier it will become to use them to create tasty, nutritious meals.

My mother told me that I should cook with herbs and that I would grow up strong and healthy—and she was right! But I do wish that she would let me choose my own swimwear!

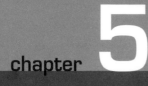

chapter **5**

Aromatic Beauty and Inner Peace

Ancient Origins

The pursuit of beauty has absorbed us for thousands of years, and it is no coincidence that some of the most impressive beauty tips are also our oldest —and simplest. Good health and beauty is not about spending a lot of money on expensive products and packaging. It's about an attitude to life and taking care of your own health. Most of the ancient beauty secrets are rooted in the sensible use of natural substances that are still available to us today.

The search for potions and lotions that bring about beauty and tranquillity is as popular today as it was centuries ago. Ancient recipes, often almost unchanged through the centuries and using mostly plant-based ingredients, abound in the herbal folklore of many different countries across the world. Each culture traditionally uses locally grown plants almost exclusively. This is largely because local plants are the most convenient ingredients available. However, it is often the active ingredients in locally grown plants that seem to resonate best with the spirit, character, and needs of the local people.

If we look at India we see that many of its beauty treatments, including the ancient Indian medical system know as Ayurveda, use ingredients such as sandalwood, turmeric, and ginger that are all grown locally. We find that sandalwood is used extensively in incense, which is used daily by most people as part of their religious rituals, in addition to being ideally suited to nourishing skin made dry by the fierce heat of the Indian sun. In less temperate countries there is much use made of indigenous herbs such as chamomile, sage, and marjoram. The gentle, warming action of marjoram provides a comforting counteraction

to cool, damp climates. Squaw vine (*Mitchella repens*) was used by many of the North American Indian tribes. It helps to prepare a woman's body for childbirth, and it was well suited to the tribal and often nomadic lifestyle of Native Americans.

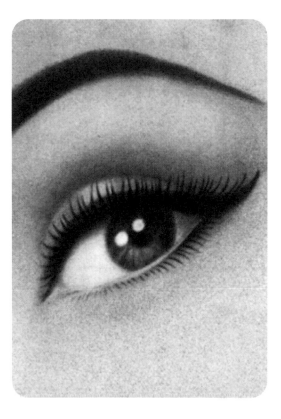

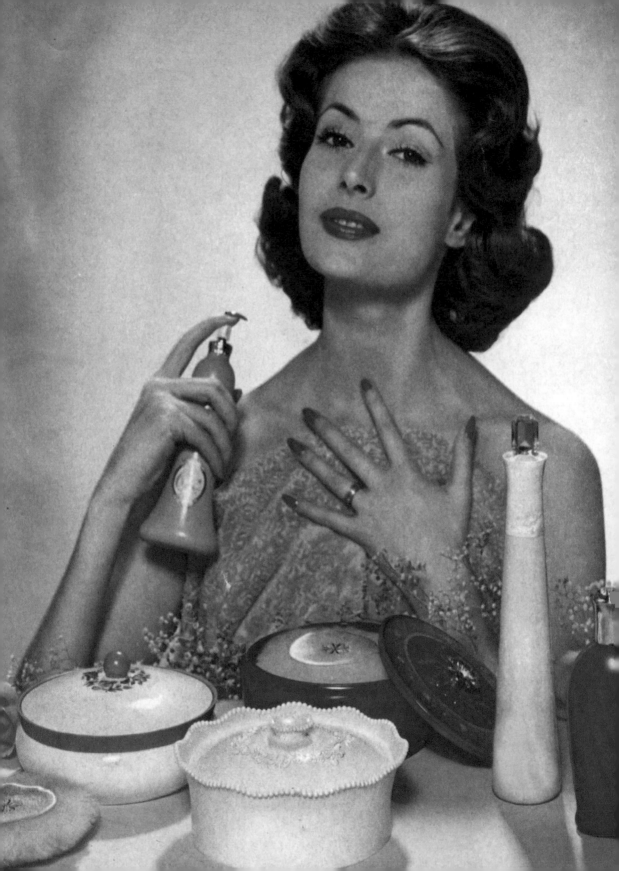

Creating your own Cosmetics

Today we have an extensive range of herbs, plants, and essential oils from around the world at our disposal. This enables us to try out many different beauty treatments, and to be able to change our cosmetic products as often as we wish. There is of course already a bewildering array of natural, plant-based beauty products stacked on the shelves of the stores. But it can be great fun to experiment with making your own personal beauty products. Armed with a few tips and safety precautions, you can easily and quickly create face creams, skin toners, bath oils, body lotions, and face packs.

One important aspect of herbal wisdom that must not be forgotten is the holistic principle. You may be aiming to create beauty treatments for external use, but to enhance their effectiveness you must also look at your lifestyle, diet, exercise, sleep patterns, and

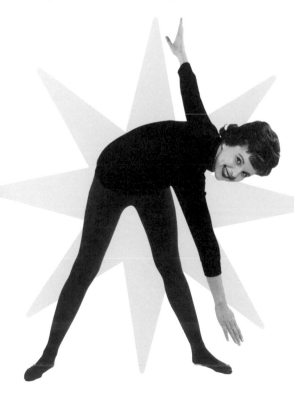

stress levels. The skin is the largest organ of the body, and if you have skin problems this is often an indication that attention needs to be given to other areas. By assessing your skin you can discover what best suits it externally, and at the same time also try to remedy the causes of any problems.

For example, because constipation prevents the effective disposal of the body's waste products, it is a common cause of blemished, dull skin and can even lead to eczema and acne—all symptomatic of a build-up of toxins in the body. Tiredness, stress, lack of exercise, and poor diet also worsen the condition of skin. Herbal treatments to help with these conditions can be found in the next chapter, and should be used alongside the following external beauty treatments when appropriate.

Facial moisturizers

This is a quick and simple recipe using essential oils and a ready-made facial-cream base. It is important to choose a base cream that is natural, unperfumed, and plant-based, so when the essential oils are mixed in they can best benefit the skin, unhindered by synthetic additives. A range of natural face creams are easily found in health food stores, herbalists, and from the retailers of natural beauty products.

Take 2oz (50g) of base face cream and place in a clean, dark glass jar. Choose your essential oil, or combination of essential oils, from the list below, always remembering that it is most important not to exceed the recommended number of drops. Stir in a total of 5 drops of essential oil thoroughly to ensure the oils are completely mixed into the cream. Use as you would any other face cream.

Dry skin: Try jasmine, chamomile, and sandalwood.

Oily skin: Geranium, lavender, and mandarin.

Sensitive skin: Use chamomile, neroli, and jasmine.

Mature skin: Try frankincense, patchouli, and rose.

Skin toners

Flowerwaters make lovely, natural, and gentle skin toners. Moisten a cotton ball with your chosen flowerwater and use as you would any other toner. Alternatively, use a spray bottle, spraying sparingly onto the face after cleansing, allowing to dry naturally before applying moisturiser.

Rosewater is best for dry, sensitive, and mature skins.

Orange Flower water is best for normal and oily skins.

Bath oils

Baths are restorative as well as cleansing. The addition of essential oils enhances the natural therapeutic effect of warm water and creates a delightful atmosphere.

Stimulating morning bath: take 4 tablespoons (60ml) of unperfumed, dispersant bath oil, pour into a dark glass bottle, and add:

10 drops of rosemary

10 drops of grapefruit

5 drops of juniper berry

5 drops of rosewood

Shake well, and use 1 teaspoon (5ml) per bath.

> ## A new way to cleanse your face

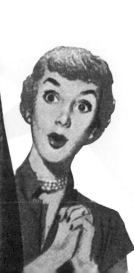

She'll prefer that "clean-groomed" look!

Relaxing, destressing evening bath: take 4 tablespoons (60ml) of natural bath oil (see bath recipe opposite) and add:

10 drops of lavender
10 drops of chamomile
5 drops of geranium
5 drops of frankincense

Shake well, and use 1 teaspoon (5ml) per bath. You can vary the proportions and essential oils as you become familiar with using them, but never exceed the total number of drops stated.

Body lotions

The addition of essential oils to unperfumed, natural body lotion not only conditions and tones the skin, but perfumes the body as well.

Exotic body lotion: (Ideal for a romantic evening!) Take 4 tablespoons (60ml) of unscented base body lotion, pour into a dark glass bottle, and add:

5 drops of sandalwood
5 drops of jasmine
5 drops of patchouli
5 drops of ylang ylang
5 drops of clary sage
5 drops of bergamot

Shake well, and use sparingly; remember that a subtle perfume is a more effective

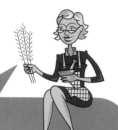

Wise Woman's Tip

It is traditional to lay slices of cucumber over the eyes while resting after a face pack has been applied. A wonderful alternative to this is to place used chamomile teabags over your eyes, but make sure they have cooled off first. Chamomile's soothing, anti-inflammatory qualities refresh tired eyes and reduce redness and soreness.

aphrodisiac than overwhelming yourself with too much scent.

After Sun body lotion: (Also good generally for dry and sensitive skin.) Take 4 tablespoons (60ml) of base body lotion as before and add:

10 drops of chamomile
5 drops of neroli
5 drops of lavender
5 drops of sandalwood

Shake the lotion well and use sparingly. If your skin needs more, use base body lotion only next, then return to the After Sun lotion again the following day.

Face packs

There is nothing like an evening spent pampering yourself and generally relaxing to restore your mind, body, and spirit. Face packs made with natural, preferably organic, ingredients may be a bit messy, but they can still be fun to prepare and use, and the benefit to your complexion makes it well worth the effort. Cleanse your face thoroughly before applying the face pack, and leave it on for between 5 and 10 minutes. After washing off

the face pack use flowerwater to tone the skin gently, and finish off with one of the moisturizers described before (whichever is best suited to your skin type).

Dry/sensitive skin: Mix ground almonds with honey to a desired consistency. Wrap your hair in a towel. Apply the pack carefully to your face, avoiding your eyes and the delicate skin surrounding them.

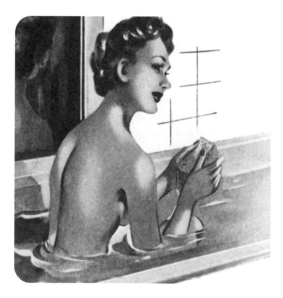

Oily skin: Mix finely ground oatmeal with natural, live yogurt to a desired consistency. Apply carefully, as before.

Normal skin: Peel and then mash an avocado to a pulp, and apply carefully as above.

Some natural beauty products

■ Aloe vera, with its cooling properties, is a good, natural external treatment for sunburn.

■ Cocoa butter has an oily consistency that melts into the skin, which makes it a very good moisturizer.

■ Oatmeal or sea salt both make excellent natural exfoliators, used in the bath or shower. Just make sure you wash down and moisturize afterwards, as sea salt especially can dry the skin.

■ Henna is a traditional, nontoxic dye for both skin and hair, though colors are limited.

■ Witchhazel has long been known for its beneficial effects on oily skin and the occasional blemish.

■ Lemon juice makes a superb hair rinse.

An appetite for beauty

What you eat can make a big difference to how you look as well as how you feel, and it's always a good idea to keep a careful eye on what you're putting into your body:

■ High-fiber foods such as brown rice and cereal help to clean out the digestive system and keep your bowels regular. This in turn helps prevent your skin from developing unwanted blemishes, or becoming dull, oversensitive or red, itchy and flaky.

■ Broccoli, carrots, and spinach are all high in vitamin A, which is believed to improve the elasticity of skin.

■ Drink lots of pure spring water—at least 6–8 glasses a day—to help flush toxins out of your body. Herbal teas are also beneficial, and better for you than black tea or coffee.

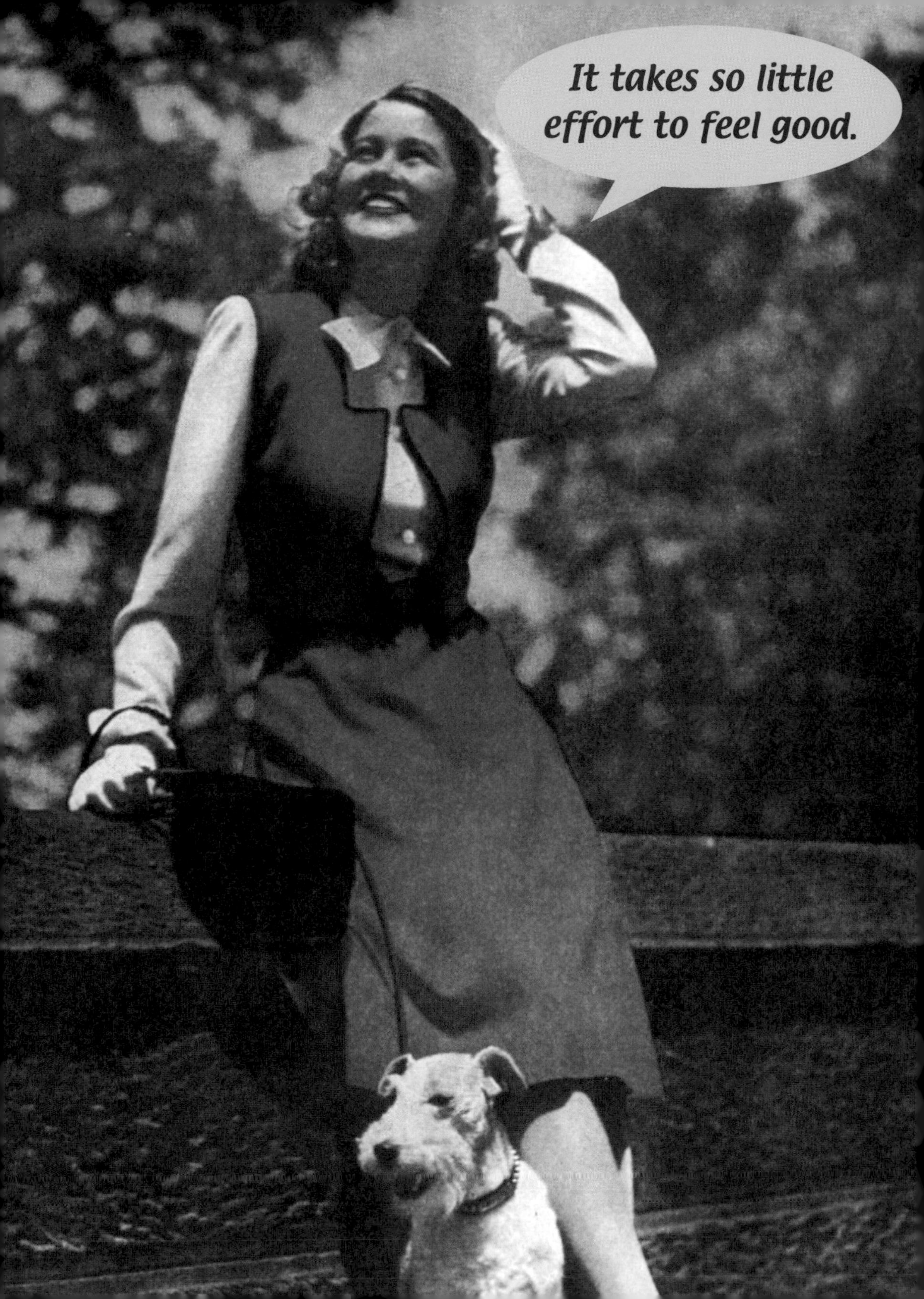
It takes so little effort to feel good.

Women's Health

This section looks at natural ways and herbal remedies to help with premenstrual tension, aches and pains, pregnancy, and menopause.

Premenstrual Tension (PMT)

The troubling symptoms of PMT are generally experienced in the week before menstruation and include: fluid retention, tender breasts, swollen or painful abdomen, irritability, mood swings, depression, and weepiness. A few lucky women never experience the monthly hormonal changes in their bodies in any debilitating way, but most women suffer from PMT, at some point in their fertile years, to a greater or lesser degree.

The first thing to check is that your PMT is not aggravated by too much ordinary stress from work and lifestyle. If at all possible, try to organize your workload to give yourself a few easier, quieter days in the week before your period starts. A healthy diet, fresh air, and exercise also play an important role in alleviating the symptoms of PMT. However, in normal life it is not always possible to look after yourself as well as you'd like. There are various herbal remedies to turn to; some were recently discovered, while others have been used throughout the ages.

Vitamin, mineral, and herbal supplements can help to alleviate PMT. The most important of these include vitamin B6 (best taken as B complex), evening primrose oil, or an herbal supplement that is rich in gamma linolenic acid (commonly known as GLA), zinc, and vitamin C. Herbal teas are helpful, especially if they are used to replace drinks high in caffeine, such as coffee and black tea. Chamomile, lemon balm, valerian, and vervain teas are relaxing, calming, and mildly sedative. If you reach the stage where everything has become too much and you feel overwhelmed, try the magic of Bach Flower Rescue Remedy. Just 5 drops in water, or even neat on the tongue, can help you regain your composure.

Certain homeopathic remedies can help with various symptoms of PMT. If the PMT is associated with tender breasts then calcarea carbonica (calc. carb.) is indicated; if feeling irritable predominates, try natrum muriaticum (nat. mur.). Weepiness can be alleviated with pulsatilla, general moodiness with sepia, and being argumentative with nux vomica (nux. vom.). A general low feeling and depression can be treated with lycopodium. As with all homeopathic self-treatment, use the sixth potency, and take 2 tablets three times a day until symptoms stop. It is a good idea to visit a qualified homeopath who can provide an in-depth assessment and specific prescription.

Menstrual cramps and other symptoms

As part of PMT, women also experience various aches and pains associated with menstruation. These include tender breasts and abdomen, headaches, bloating, and fluid retention. Evening primrose oil and vitamins B6 can help to prevent these symptoms, but if they do still occur various herbs can alleviate them. Red raspberry leaf tea is a well-known remedy for menstrual cramps. Before and during your period, infuse the tea for 10 minutes in boiling water and drink one cup two or three times a day. Or try cramp bark (Viburnum opulus) mixed in equal parts with chamomile and a slice of ginger root and infused for 10 minutes in boiling water. A hot compress over the abdomen with essential oils of marjoram and clary sage is comforting and alleviates cramps and pain.

Fluid retention, which produces a general bloated feeling, can be relieved by gentle herbal diuretics such as dandelion and chamomile. Reducing caffeine, alcohol, and other toxins and replacing them with infusions of dandelion and chamomile can substantially reduce the discomfort. Rest and relaxation are important. Set aside time to relax by taking an aromatic bath with essential oils of lavender and clary sage. Use a total of 5 drops of these two oils mixed into 1 teaspoon (5ml) of dispersant base bath oil in a warm, not overly hot, bath. The homeopathic remedy graphites can be useful to counteract a bloated, heavy feeling, particularly if weight gain is experienced.

Pregnancy

This is a very special time in a woman's life, especially with a first child, and heralds a major life-changing situation. This brings up a range of feelings and emotions as well as dramatic physical changes as the baby grows and develops. A good way to deal with these physical, hormonal, and emotional changes is to create as much space and time as possible to nest—just like birds and animals. Try to stay in touch with the miracle of reproduction as it is happening moment by moment.

Medicines, herbal and allopathic, should be kept to an absolute minimum during pregnancy because everything the mother ingests affects the baby. However, mild, gentle herbal teas are fine, and can help to reduce caffeine intake. In the later stages the herb that stands out as the expectant mother's greatest friend is raspberry leaf. It has an excellent reputation from herbal folklore, and is still recommended by modern herbalists. Raspberry leaf tones and strengthens the whole reproductive system and prepares the mother for giving birth. It is best taken as a tea, with three cups a day drunk at regular intervals. Various forms of raspberry leaf extract are available from health food stores if you don't want to drink the tea itself.

Morning sickness

This can sometimes be prevented by keeping to a good, nutritious diet. Junk food laden with fat, salt, sugar, chemicals, and additives must be avoided. Vitamin supplements tailored to the pregnant woman's needs can also be taken. Nonetheless, sometimes morning

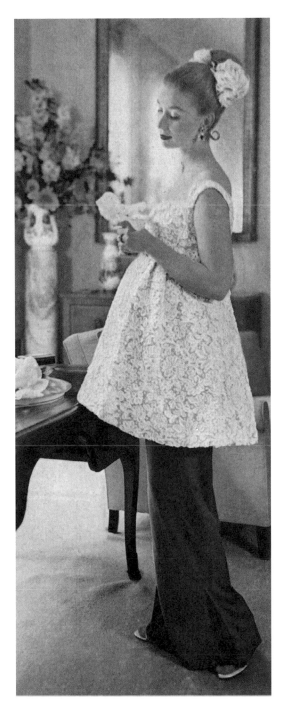

hormones and sometimes to the anticlimax felt after childbirth. This is called postpartum or postnatal depression. If symptoms are severe, then it is necessary to consult your doctor first, and then a qualified medical herbalist. However, it is common to feel a sense of anticlimax and general low spirits as the reality of caring for a small baby hits home. Often this is aggravated by the new mother being so busy caring for her baby that she neglects to feed herself properly and at the same time is suffering from lack of sleep. Vitamin B deficiency is not uncommon, and a B complex supplement or a strengthening herbal tonic can be taken. Oats are both nourishing and a tonic to the nerves and should be included in the diet.

Fennel tea assists the flow of breast milk, and raspberry leaf tea helps the tired uterine muscles recover from birth. Lemon balm, vervain, and chamomile teas can all help with mild depression, as can an infusion of catnip. A tiny dab of rose essential oil behind the ears and on the inside of the wrists will lift the spirits. Rose is also a uterine tonic.

sickness will still strike down the healthiest of women. Peppermint tea drunk first thing in the morning is often successful at alleviating symptoms. Chamomile tea is a good alternative. An infusion of meadowsweet or chopped fresh ginger root—sweetened with a little honey if desired—can be very helpful.

Postpartum depression

It is not uncommon to experience depression after giving birth, due to wildly fluctuating

Menopause

This can be a challenging time for women, as much psychologically as hormonally. The sense of loss of fertility, the vital essence of being a woman, needs to be grieved for at the same time as coping with sometimes substantial physical changes to the body. Most notable and often distressing are the hot flashes caused by the rush of hormones into the blood as the gland system gradually adjusts to the new situation. Other symptoms include irregular periods that gradually lessen until they disappear, depression, and mood swings.

The berries of the chaste tree *(Vitex agnus-castus)* are used to normalize the hormonal changes associated with menopause. Traditionally, an infusion was made with the ripe berries, but a selection of ready-made agnus castus herbal treatments from health food stores and herbalists are available.

Other useful herbs that can be combined with chaste berry are wild yam, black cohosh, golden seal and motherwort. If serious depression is experienced while going through menopause, see your doctor. However, mild depression can be helped by skullcap, valerian, and St. John's Wort. These can be bought as dried herbs individually, or as a mixture from an herbalist. An infusion should be drunk two or three times a day. There are also mixed herbal teas specifically designed for menopausal women, and St. John's Wort is available as a tincture, which is quick and easy to take in water.

Other general tips for dealing with the menopause:

■ Lifestyle and activity can influence the severity of some symptoms you experience. Women who exercise regularly are less likely to develop osteoporosis.

■ Plant estrogens found in soy, flax seed, and other plants can help to balance hormones.

■ The risk of developing heart disease increases after the menopause, so it becomes even more important to follow a low-cholesterol diet.

■ It is thought that vitamin E, found in nuts, wheatgerm, and avocados, reduces the impact of hot flashes.

General good health

While there are several specific health issues that affect women and need their own treatment, you should always take good day-to-day care of your

Wise Woman's Tip

Research has discovered that soy-rich foods, such as tofu and soymilk, as well as yams, squash, and carrots, contain plant estrogens, called phytoestrogens. Asian women, whose diet is abundant in soy, report a far lower incidence of hot flashes during menopause. So stock up on your soy!

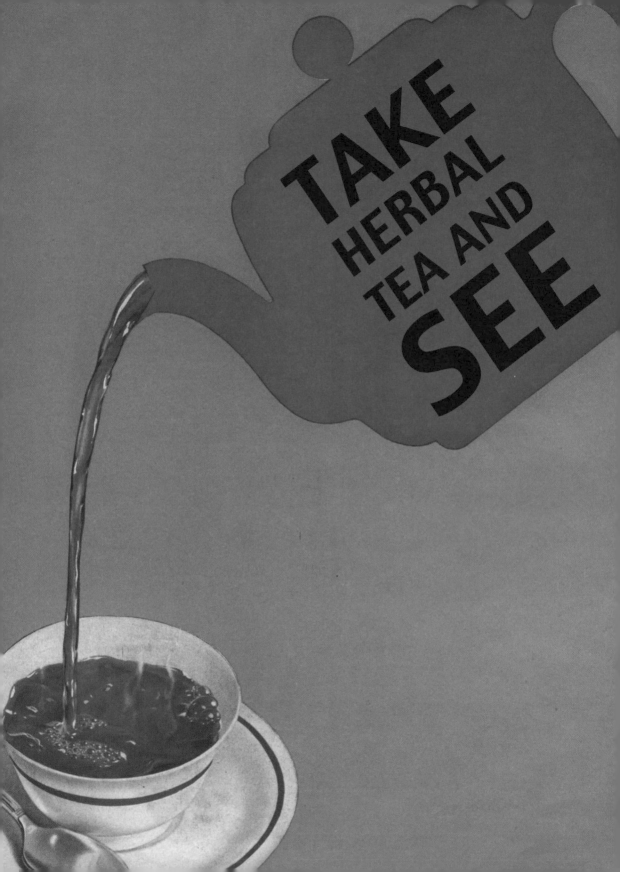

health. There are a number of ways in which women can look after their general well-being:

■ Adopt a gentle keep-fit program such as yoga or tai chi. These exercise programs gently stretch the body and also engage the mind, making them a good way of looking after both your physical and emotional health.

■ Remember to take time off. Just half an hour's rest and relaxation at the end of a busy day can make all the difference. Have a long soak in the bath or practice breathing exercises. Have an early night and get enough sleep, then you will feel refreshed in the morning. You will feel so much better in the morning.

■ Keep an eye on your eating habits. Too much dairy produce, alcohol, or caffeine can have a detrimental effect. What our grand-parents said still rings true: everything in moderation. Don't stop giving yourself occasional treats, just remember to eat healthy foods, too.

■ A healthy mental and emotional state positively affects your physical health. Try to keep mentally active with hobbies and interests, and try meditation to facilitate a tranquil mind.

Inner Peace

The natural remedies and beauty treatments described earlier promote health, well-being, and outer beauty. They can be complemented by using essential oils for self-massage, and by burning essential oils during meditation to discover the beauty inside, the tranquility of inner peace.

Self-massage

Although it is a lovely treat to receive a massage from a fully trained aromatherapist or other massage therapist, there are many benefits in massaging yourself using essential oils. Self-massage is a strong natural instinct. We use it when we bump ourselves, for instance, rubbing the painful area better. Self-massage is also empowering and can bring a sense of positively caring for yourself with the comfort and reassurance of your own nurturing touch. The feeling of well-being provided by self-massage is a link between the body, the emotions, and the inner spirit or soul. Regular self-massage unites these different parts of yourself and heals pain, tension, and stress, leading you toward inner peace.

Using essential oils

Incorporating the healing power of essential oils improves the benefits of self-massage enormously, and promotes a feeling of inner well-being and peace. Aromatic herbs, flowers, woods, and spices have been used in this way for centuries. Our ancestors made simple infused oils by steeping aromatic plant materials in oil or animal fat, but today, blending essential oils into a base oil is a quicker and more convenient way to harness the magic of aromatic plants. To make sufficient massage oil for a self-massage, take 1 tablespoon (15ml) of almond or sunflower oil and thoroughly mix in up to, but not exceeding, a total of 9 drops of essential oil.

Many essential oils can be used in self-massage, so personal likes and dislikes are important when making a selection. Surrounding yourself with a scent you dislike will not be of much benefit, whereas being drawn naturally to certain aromas is your body's way of telling you which oils will work well for you. Experiment with different oils to discover which individual oils and blends suit you best. The following list includes some of the most effective essential oils that promote relaxation and inner peace. Try a self-massage with a blend of two oils, and then experiment with three or four.

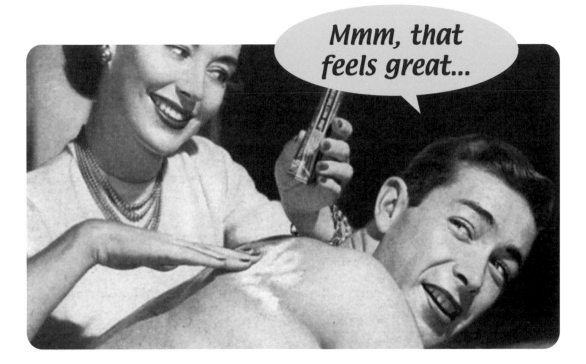

■ **Frankincense:** A traditional ingredient of incense with a strong spiritual vibration. It has a tonic effect on the respiratory system and slows down the breathing.

■ **Marjoram:** Warming, soothing, and comforting, marjoram supports the personal quest for inner peace.

■ **Chamomile:** Cooling and comforting, chamomile helps you to leave stress and tension behind (you've probably tried the tea).

■ **Lavender:** This oil provides a calm, tranquil aroma that is deeply relaxing and refreshing.

■ **Rose:** A most delightful sweet scent that provides a comfort zone beyond the trials and tribulations of daily life.

■ **Geranium:** This oil balances mind, body, and spirit, helping you to find equilibrium.

■ **Rosewood:** Soft but powerful, rosewood helps you to connect with your spiritual center.

Create a quiet, warm, private space, undress to your underwear, and make sure you have enough towels to keep yourself warm and to protect clothing. Pour a little oil onto your hands and with long, firm strokes massage up your legs, first one leg then the other. Notice the different sensations, what feels good and what doesn't, and adjust the firmness and technique of your massage strokes accordingly. Try to cover as much of your legs as possible, front and back, from ankle to hip. Then move onto your arms, including the shoulders. Shoulders always carry a lot of tension so knead the muscles well, going as deep as feels comfortable. If you have any oil left and your hands are not tired, you can finish by lying on your back and massaging your abdomen gently in a clockwise direction. If all this sounds like too much work, you can make up less massage oil and just give yourself a foot massage.

Meditation

Aromatic plants have been used extensively to aid meditation and religious rituals throughout the ages. Frankincense is still burned in Roman Catholic churches as an integral part of the religious ceremony. Other religions burn incense during their rituals in temples, and as offerings. The incense they use contains different aromatics, many of which are derived from plants. As well as frankincense, traditional ingredients of incense include juniper, cedarwood, sandalwood, cypress, and myrrh. Mary anointed the feet of Jesus with spikenard, and according to some authorities the name of Gethsemane was a version of jessamine or jasmine. These examples clearly demonstrate the importance of aromatic plants in spiritual rituals throughout the ages.

When we meditate we discover inner peace and happiness and also feel better because meditation enhances healing and good health. When you meditate you become aware of what it feels like to be alive by focusing on your breathing and physical sensations as they arise and pass throughout the body. Most of our lives are spent rushing around doing things; meditation is about discovering what it means to be a human being.

Meditation is a powerful method for self-discovery, an internal process of becoming familiar with your mind and the thoughts that endlessly tumble through it. By watching your breath come and go and your thoughts arise and pass you develop an inner knowledge that living, being alive, is an ever-changing process. We are not static entities, we change subtly moment by moment. This inner knowledge helps you to accept the natural flow of life, and find a deep, inner peace in the here and now, beyond the hectic schedule of daily life.

Burning incense and essential oils

The simplest way to use aromatic plants with meditation is to burn incense. There are many commercial brands available, and some incense is specifically designed to promote healing. This includes some Tibetan incense that contains ingredients also used in Tibetan medicine, a highly sophisticated system that utilizes many herbs and other aromatics. When choosing incense make sure you like the smell before buying and burning it. Most incense is very powerful, and it is important to feel comfortable with the aroma so the incense is an aid to meditation, not an unpleasant distraction.

If you have an essential-oil burner, you can choose to burn essential oils instead. Place a lighted tea-light under the ceramic bowl already filled with hot water. Sprinkle a few drops of your chosen essential oil on top; it will start to evaporate with the heat. This method allows you to be very specific with the aroma you wish to introduce to assist your

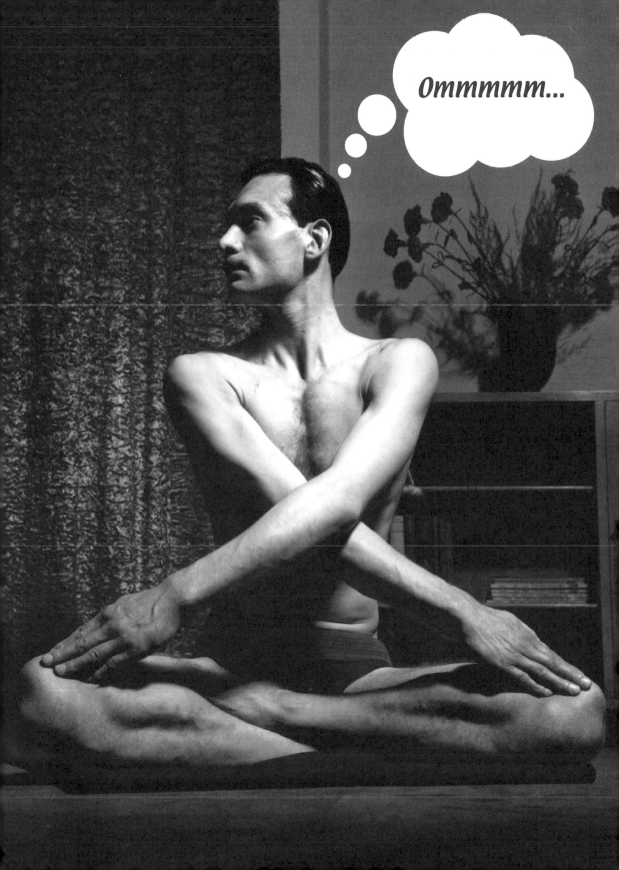

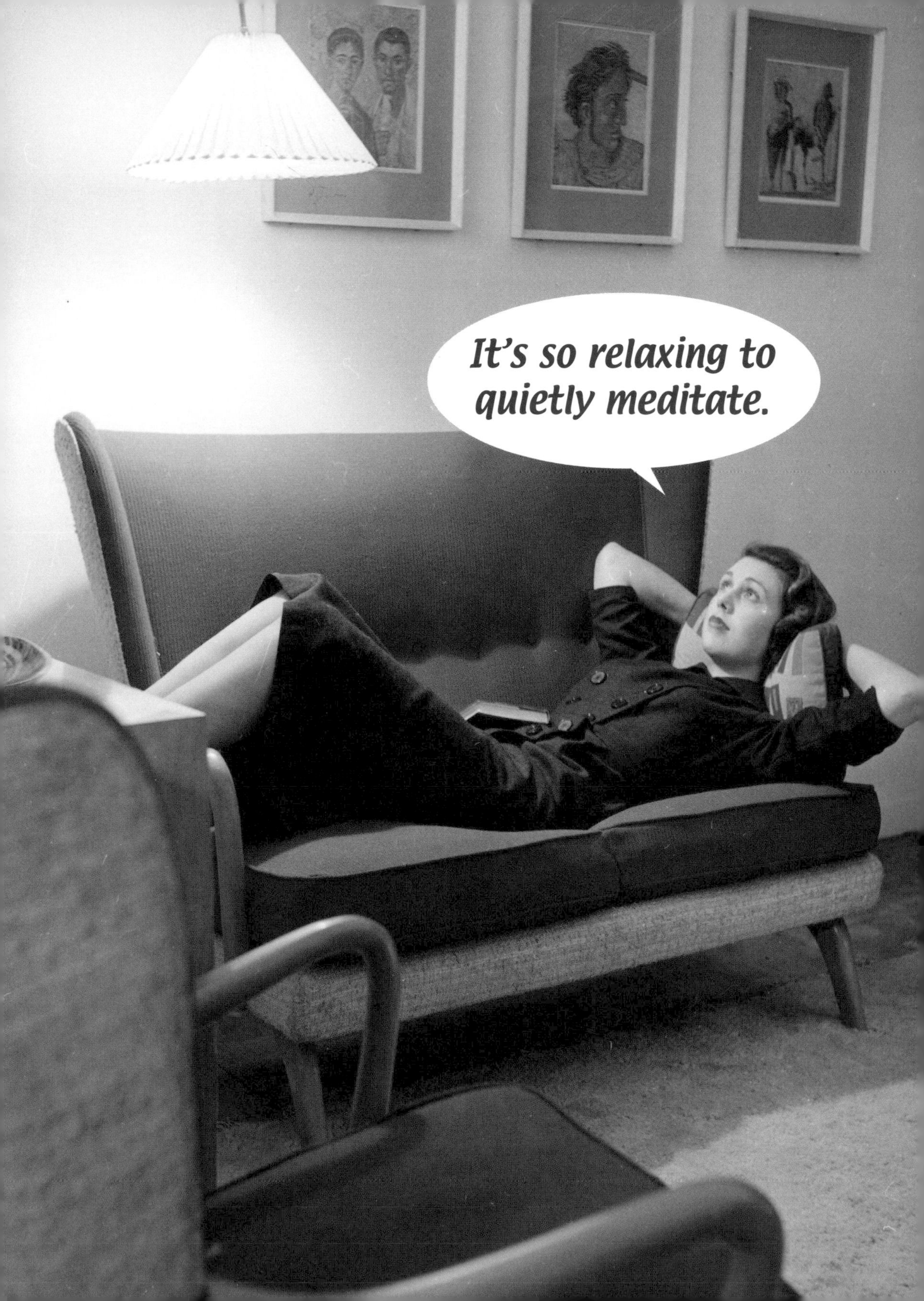
It's so relaxing to quietly meditate.

meditation, rather than relying on a premixed incense. It also allows you to choose essential oils that can help with physical ailments, so if, for instance, you have a headache, burning lavender as you meditate will also help to relieve the headache.

How to meditate

First, find somewhere private where you will not be disturbed. Disconnect the telephone or put it onto the answering machine. Light your incense or prepare your essential-oil burner as described above. Then sit comfortably cross-legged on a cushion on the floor, or up on a chair with both feet flat on the floor. Meditation is best done with a straight back, which allows the body's energies to flow freely. Keep the eyes lightly closed with your hands resting on your knees.

Bring your attention to your breathing and feel the sensations of your breath entering and leaving your body—at the tip of the nostrils, or the rising and falling of the abdomen. Be aware of the scent of the incense or essential oils.

As you continue watching your breath, observe how thoughts come into your mind. Instead of just thinking all your thoughts, try to acknowledge each one as just a thought and then let it go. Don't worry if you can't do it; it takes many years of dedicated meditation to be able to let your thoughts pass without succumbing to thinking some of them. But even the attempt is a form of meditation, and it will gradually bring peace and quiet to the mind, body, and spirit.

Allow 5–10 minutes when you first start, then meditate for longer if you wish, once you gain some experience. Meditation is most effective if it is done regularly, daily if possible. You can experiment with different incenses and oils and observe how they can influence your moods.

6

Natural First-Aid Remedies

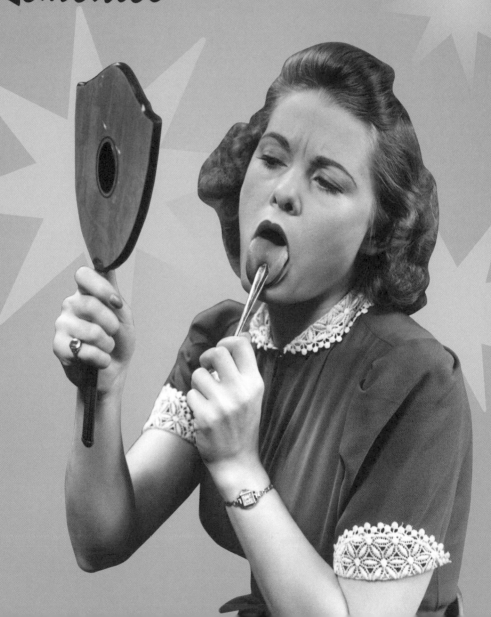

What Treatments Should I Take?

The suggestions given here are for first aid and to treat mild conditions only. If symptoms do not improve, or the condition is, or becomes serious, seek medical advice immediately because it would be dangerous to try self-diagnosis and self-treatment. However, the natural remedies described here can certainly help minor ailments and accidents, and have been successfully used for many years.

Asthma

During an asthma attack take some Rescue Remedy, and sit quietly and sniff lavender, frankincense, bergamot, or chamomile essential oils either directly from the bottle or from a tissue with a few drops sprinkled on. Do not use steam inhalation as the heat could aggravate the condition. Moisture is beneficial though, and a humidifier or room spray can be used with plain water or a few drops of essential oil added. To try to lessen the severity and frequency of attacks, try daily yoga exercises to open the chest and deepen the breathing, and massage the upper back and chest with any of the essential oils mentioned above in 3% dilution. Proprietary herbal remedies are available to take when feeling susceptible to an attack; those containing lobelia are thought to be particularly effective.

Athlete's foot

This irritating, and common, fungal infection between the toes responds well to antifungal essential oils, especially tea tree, myrrh, and lavender. Dilute 3 drops of any of these essential oils, singly or mixed, into 1 teaspoon (5ml) of vodka, and use this to swab the affected area. After a few days, when the

condition has improved, switch to calendula cream with the same proportion of essential oils mixed in. Keep the feet scrupulously clean to discourage the fungal infection. If you are

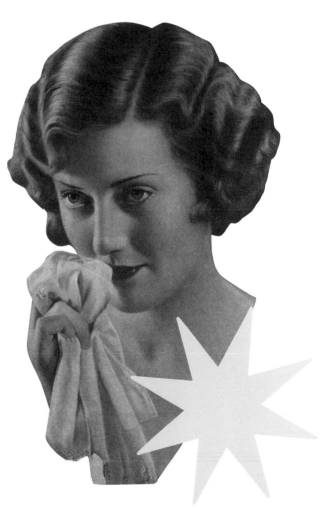

prone to athlete's foot, ensure that you wear only cotton socks, let your feet breathe free from footwear for some time every day, and avoid synthetic running shoes.

Bronchitis and coughs

When bronchitis strikes and also brings loss of voice or hoarseness, take the homeopathic remedy phosphorus. The essential oils of

benzoin, bergamot, sandalwood, and thyme all have expectorant qualities and one or more of these should be used in steam inhalations, in the bath, and in local massage to the upper back and chest. Moisture also helps coughs and bronchitis, and the affected person should rest in a warm room in which a kettle is regularly boiled, or should use a humidifier, until the symptoms ease off. Make a

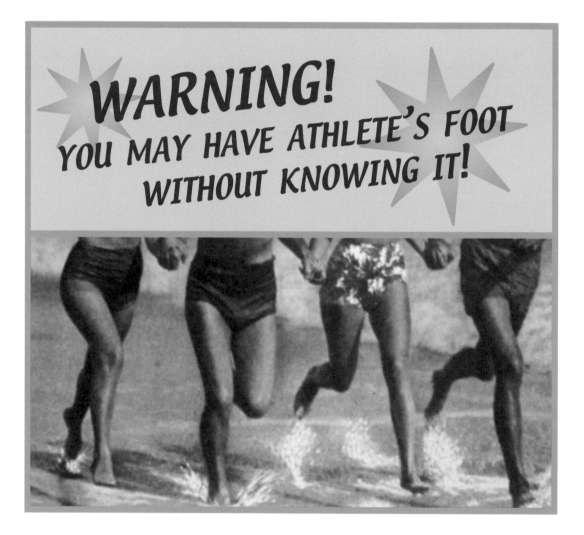

Cough...cough ...cough!

decoction using elecampane and licorice roots, and mix this into an infusion of white horehound and marshmallow—drink a warm cupful three times a day. Fresh ginger is also helpful, and a decoction of ginger with fresh lemon and honey can be drunk when desired. Take one garlic capsule twice a day, and drink some homemade onion soup. If the bronchitis worsens or a fever develops, visit a doctor immediately.

Bruises

Take arnica homeopathic tablets as soon as possible after the bruising occurs. Use an ice-cold compress of witch hazel to reduce the pain and swelling, and then apply arnica ointment if the skin is unbroken, or comfrey ointment if the skin is broken. If the bruise is still painful at bedtime, add 3 drops of lavender oil to comfrey or calendula ointment and smooth over the bruise.

Burns

The most important action is to immediately cool the burn by plunging the affected part in cold water and leaving it there for at least 5 minutes. If immersing the body part is not possible, then soak a large towel with cold water and apply it to the burn, moving the towel frequently to keep the coldest part in contact with the burn. Take Rescue Remedy and arnica to counteract the shock, and take cantharis homeopathic tablets once the immediate situation has been resolved. There are several good natural treatments for minor burns, the most effective of which is lavender essential oil. This is one of the few occasions when the oil is applied neat to the skin. Gently cover the burn with lavender oil, and repeat if necessary after half an hour. However, lavender often works magically to heal minor burns and subdue the pain with just one application. Alternatives, if you do not have lavender oil, are honey, calendula ointment, or cold compresses of cooled chamomile tea. (See also Shock, on page 136.)

Colds

You might be able to prevent a cold by taking echinacea drops and aconite homeopathic tablets at the first signs of a cold. Should symptoms develop, drink an infusion of elderflower tea and start doing steam inhalations with lavender, eucalyptus, and tea tree. Go to bed early with an infusion of fresh ginger, lemon juice, and honey, and wrap up warm to encourage sweating. A burner of lavender essential oil will help to fight infection, prevent others in the household from catching the cold, and aid a good night's sleep (be sure to extinguish the candle in the burner before you go to sleep). A tissue with a few drops of eucalyptus oil can be kept at hand to help clear a stuffy nose. Eat lots of onions and garlic, or take garlic capsules if you dislike the taste of garlic, and drink lots of fluids, especially chamomile, elderflower, or peppermint teas.

Cold sores

These are caused by the herpes simplex 1 virus, and tend to appear when you are run down, or have a cold or other infection. Take echinacea to boost your immune system. Use essential oils of bergamot, lavender, or tea tree diluted in vodka, using 6 drops to 1 teaspoon (5ml) of vodka and dab on frequently. Tea tree gel is a good alternative, as is tincture of calendula.

Conjunctivitis and sore eyes

Conjunctivitis is a bacterial infection, so wash hands before and after touching the eyes. Sterilize the eye-bath you will use with boiling water and use a separate batch of lotion for each eye to prevent cross-infection. Use any of the following as a soothing eyewash, several times a day: cooled infusion of chamomile or elderflower, 2 drops of euphrasia in cooled boiled water, with the addition of a few drops of rosewater if desired. Take argentum nitricum or euphrasia homeopathic tablets.

Constipation

Improving your diet by eliminating refined carbohydrates and increasing fiber, fresh fruit, and vegetables helps to normalize the colon and bowel functions. Drinking lots of water and herb teas is recommended, as is eating figs and prunes and increasing your daily

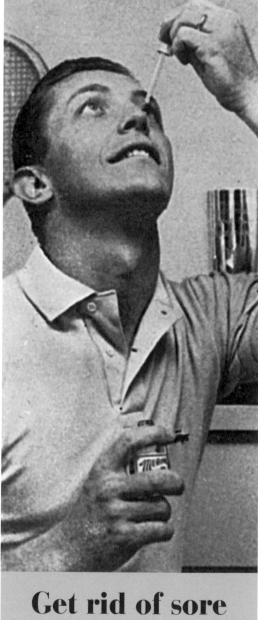

Get rid of sore eyes—fast!

exercise. For immediate relief, massage your abdomen in a clockwise direction using 2 drops of marjoram and 1 drop of black pepper essential oils in 1 teaspoon (5ml) of almond oil. Certain yoga exercises strengthen and tone the muscles of the abdomen. The homeopathic remedies of nux. vom. and sulfur can also help to relieve the problem. Drink an infusion of senna, or any natural herbal constipation tonic, to combat occasional bouts of constipation, but do not use these regularly because in the long term they prove counterproductive.

Convalescence

It is essential to rest and regain strength after illness. Good nutrition is important and oats are a natural tonic. The following supplements all help the body regain its strength—choose from a weekly course of Ginseng, Floradix™, royal jelly, or aloe vera. An infusion of vervain, drunk three times a day, is also helpful.

Cuts and grazes

Take arnica or hypericum homeopathic tablets and see also Shock, below. Cuts and grazes should first be washed carefully to remove all dirt. Add a couple of drops of tea tree or lemon essential oils, or tincture of calendula, to a bowl of warm water and swab the area gently with a cotton ball soaked in the water. Then apply comfrey ointment to the cut and dress lightly with a sterilized dressing. Check every day, and as soon as possible leave the cut to the open air to speed healing. You can continue using comfrey ointment or calendula at this point if you like.

Cystitis

Take cantharis homeopathic tablets, and drink lots of water and chamomile tea at the first signs of cystitis. Make a decoction of marshmallow root, and drink a cupful three times a day. Garlic capsules should be taken orally, and also used as a suppository placed up the rectum after a bowel movement. Use essential oils of bergamot and tea tree as a local wash, a total of 3 drops per 1 pint (500ml) of water, well shaken each time before using. Baths with tea tree, lavender, or chamomile oils will help. If there is pain and anxiety, take Rescue Remedy, and use a hot compress of bergamot, chamomile, and sandalwood oils over the abdomen. If the

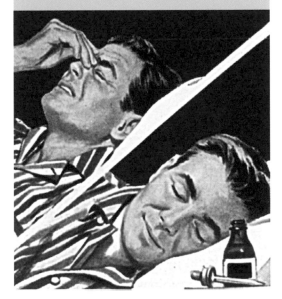

When your nose fills up at night...

Here's to the joy of glowing health!

GRAPEFRUIT JUICE OFFERS ALL THIS HELP TO HEALTH EACH DAY!

1. Helps maintain alkaline reserve

2. Supplies liquid hostile to colds

3. A gold mine of vitamin C

4. Other vitamins and minerals

5. Energy from fruit sugars

6. Arouses sulky appetites

7. Stimulates digestive juices so mildly laxative

discomfort increases or there is blood or pus in the urine, see a doctor immediately.

Diarrhea

If this is brought on by nerves or fear such as before an exam or interview, take Rescue Remedy, the homeopathic remedy argentum nitricum, and sniff essential oil of neroli to calm the nerves. If the diarrhea is from food poisoning or a digestive upset, take arsenicum album homeopathic tablets. Avoid fruit until the symptoms have passed, except raw grated apple, which helps to absorb excess moisture, as do porridge oats. Make an infusion of equal parts agrimony and meadowsweet, sweeten with honey, and drink a cupful every two hours. A decoction of cinnamon sweetened with honey is an alternative, as is peppermint tea.

Digestive problems

There are a variety of mild digestive problems such as gas and wind, heartburn, nausea, indigestion, and colic. Often these are brought on by a rich meal, eating too much, or a generally poor diet. If you are prone to any of these, try to improve and simplify your diet for a month, and include as many of the culinary herbs mentioned previously as possible. This alone may well relieve the symptoms. Meanwhile, for gas and wind try a cupful of fennel tea after meals, or a decoction of cinnamon, cloves, nutmeg, or cardamom taken in a little warm milk sweetened with honey. Nausea and colic can be relieved with peppermint, chamomile, lemon balm, or ginger tea, cinnamon in milk, or a decoction of

slippery elm. For indigestion and acidity, try any of the herbal teas above, or an infusion of meadowsweet. Decoctions of cinnamon, nutmeg, anise, or cardamom sweetened with honey will also help.

Earaches

Take the homeopathic remedy belladonna, and apply hot compresses of lavender and chamomile to the outside of the ear and its immediate surrounding area. It is important to seek a doctor's advice if the condition worsens. Avoid sticking anything in the ear —this might aggravate a possible infection.

Eczema and skin problems

Eczema is usually aggravated by stress and nervous tension, and this must be treated alongside the eczema. The symptoms of red, itchy, flaky skin are similar to allergic reactions and dermatitis and the following treatments are suitable for all these skin conditions. Avoid wearing synthetic material next to the skin, and avoid highly perfumed soaps and skin creams; also use nonbiological laundry detergent. Occasionally this type of skin condition reflects a disorder in the internal organs, and could be caused by a toxic overload in the liver. If you think this might be the cause, pay a visit to an acupuncturist; as acupuncture is an excellent treatment for such cases. Aromatherapy massage helps to relieve stress and tension, and this can be supplemented by using essential oils of chamomile, geranium, or lavender in the bath. Make chamomile tea to drink, and use the chilled tea bags as a cold compress on

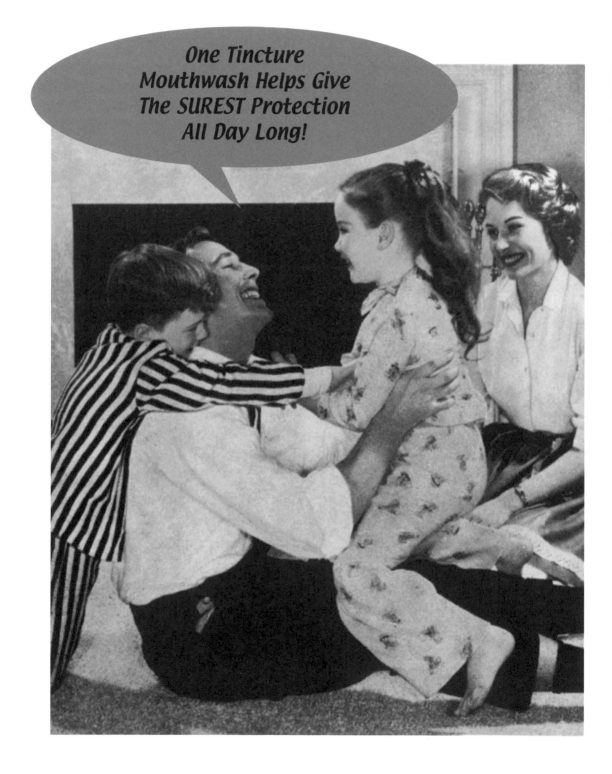

patches of affected skin. A body lotion with a 1% dilution (1 drop per teaspoon/5ml) of chamomile and melissa essential oils can be applied twice a day. A daily supplement of evening primrose oil is recommended.

Fever

Mild fevers are the body's way of dealing with infection and toxic wastes. The sweating that accompanies fever is part of the healing process and should not be suppressed. If the fever is serious, seek medical attention immediately. Drinking hot herbal infusions helps to promote sweating, and the patient should be in a warm bed in a well ventilated room. Peppermint, yarrow, elderflower, and lemon balm are all recommended, either singly or in combination.

Gum problems

Gingivitis is an inflammation of the gums causing soreness and bleeding. Take the homeopathic remedy calcarea phosphorica, and echinacea and vitamin C to boost your immune system. Take a tincture of myrrh, thyme, sage, or fennel, 6 drops in a cup of hot water, and use as a mouthwash, swishing it around in your mouth for 5–10 minutes four times a day. Check that you are using your toothbrush correctly, and buy a new one if necessary. If the condition does not clear or improve in a few days, visit your dentist.

Hemorrhoids

The wonderfully named pilewort (*Ranunculus ficarai*), also know as lesser celandine, is the classic herbal remedy for hemorrhoids. It is

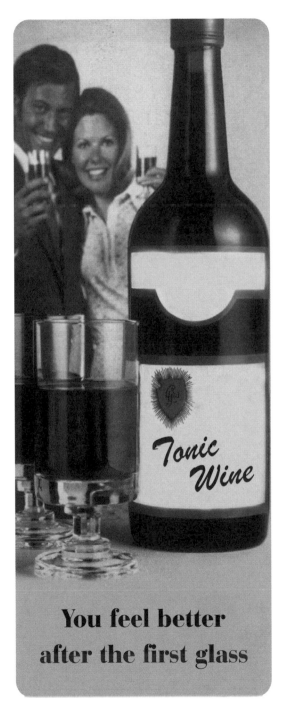

You feel better
after the first glass

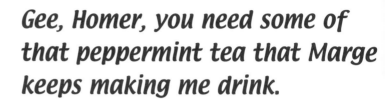

easiest to purchase a natural herbal ointment containing pilewort, however a tincture made from the dried root could be mixed into calendula ointment, together with tincture of agrimony. If the piles are sensitive the homeopathic remedy hypericum is recommended; if there is itching use nux vom. Essential oil of cypress can be used instead of pilewort if preferred, mixed into calendula ointment, at a ratio of 3 drops to 1 teaspoon (5ml).

Hangovers

As well as a throbbing headache and nausea, your liver is also suffering if you have imbibed too much alcohol. A glass of warm water with the juice of half a lemon will help to detoxify the liver. Drink this and lie in a darkened room for half an hour. Then drink a cup of an herbal infusion made from peppermint, lime flowers, lavender, and rosemary, which should provide further relief. Eat bananas and drink as much water as possible. A couple of drops of lavender essential oil rubbed on the temples will help the headache, and if it is really bad, try a cold compress with lavender. Other than abstinence, the best cure is prevention. Take 1 gram of vitamin C and drink a pint of water before going to bed after a night out and this should make the hangover much less severe.

Hay fever (Allergic rhinitis)

Take the homeopathic tablets euphrasia and use the liquid as an eyewash, 2 drops in an eyebath of warm water, every few hours. Drink an infusion of chamomile and lemon balm, and sprinkle a few drops of chamomile essential oil

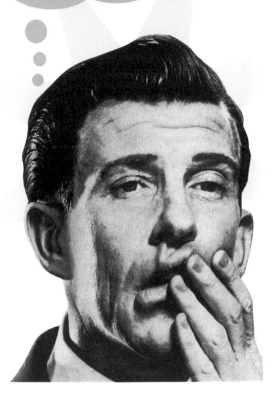

Oooh, my hangover...

onto a tissue and sniff frequently. Ice-cold rosewater or witch hazel can be used as a cold compress over the eyes and nose.

Headaches

A cold compress using essential oils of lavender and peppermint, applied to the forehead, is recommended, preferably with the patient lying down in a darkened room for half an hour. Massage the neck with essential oil of marjoram, 3 drops in 1 teaspoon (5ml) of almond oil. Drink an infusion of lime flower, chamomile, and lavender, sweetened with

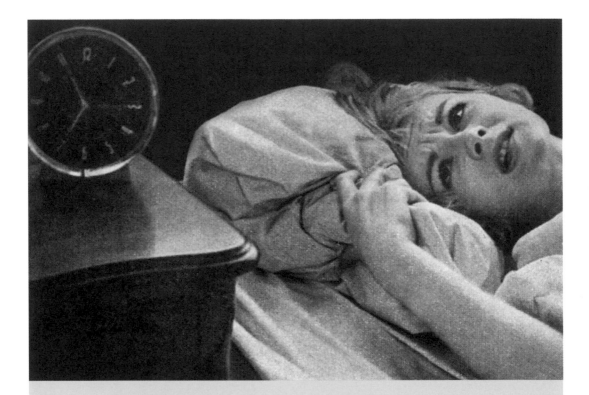

Don't let flu get you down

honey if desired. Headaches are often caused by stress and tension so it is a good idea to take some time out for relaxation if this is the cause (see also Stress).

Influenza

One of the best herbs for the relief of influenza is boneset (*Eupatorium perfoliatum*). A cup of an infusion of boneset, with elderflowers and peppermint if desired, should be drunk as often as possible for as long as the symptoms

last. When influenza strikes it is best to give in to the debility and rest in bed, sleeping as much as possible. Once the symptoms start to clear, take an herbal tonic such as Floradix™, or take ginseng or royal jelly. Prevention is better than cure, so if you feel you are coming down with the flu, take echinacea and have a bath with 3 drops each of lavender and tea tree essential oils mixed into 1 teaspoon (5ml) of base bath oil, and go to bed immediately afterward. These essential oils diffused in a burner in the sick room will help the patient and also help those who are caring for them to avoid catching the virus.

Insect bites and stings

Make sure you get the sting out if possible. Then apply an ice-cold compress of witch hazel, until the immediate pain has eased. If none is available, rub the juice and zest of a lemon over the sting, or a raw onion if you don't mind the smell. Apply a couple of drops of lavender essential oil, tea tree gel, or tincture of calendula. Take apis mellifica homeopathic tablets.

Insomnia

There is a wealth of natural, herbal remedies to counteract insomnia, but it is important not to develop a dependency on any of them. This is not because they are addictive, but that long-term use will gradually impair the body's own natural mechanisms for going to sleep. Occasional use will, however, dispel the odd night's sleeplessness. There are proprietary brands of herbal teas, which are pleasant mixes of various sleep-promoting herbs. If you prefer to make your own infusion, choose from chamomile, lime flower, vervain, lemon balm, passionflower, valerian, and hops. Any of these, singly or in combination will help bring about a good night's sleep. A couple of drops of lavender essential oil on the pillow will also help. Avoid caffeine from mid-afternoon onwards.

Laryngitis and sore throats

Doing regular steam inhalations with Friar's Balsam or essential oils of thyme, rosewood,

sandalwood, or lavender is the first choice to treat sore throats. This can be supplemented with regular gargling using tincture of thyme or sage, 6 drops in a cup of warm water, and an infusion of these herbs together with chamomile can be drunk as well.

Nervous tension and stress

The best way to deal with these conditions is to try to deal with the causes, and reduce the factors that are leading to nervous tension and stress in the first place. Of course, it is not always possible to remove all the factors, so learning how to cope with the resulting tension is important. Take time out to meditate, practice yoga or tai chi, or even just take a walk to help alleviate stress. Reducing caffeine and substituting herbal teas is also helpful. Valerian is the classic herbal remedy, but it tastes horrible on its own. It can, however, be successfully combined with any of

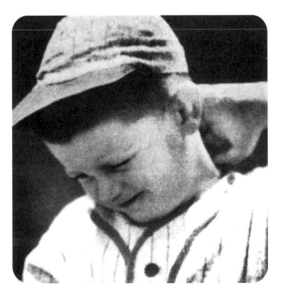

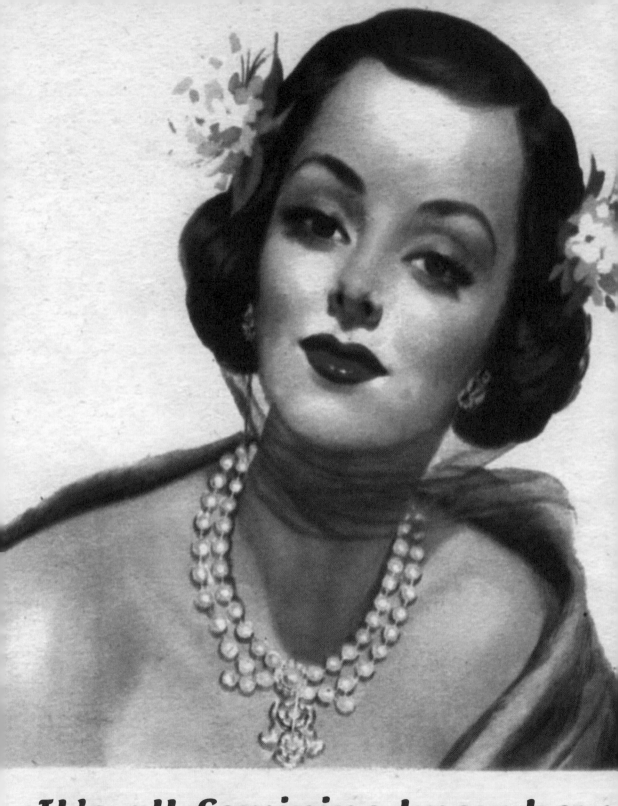

It's all feminine know-how

the following: chamomile, vervain, lime flower, lemon balm, skullcap, hops, and passionflower with honey added to sweeten it. Or there are proprietary herbal tablets for nerves containing valerian, which can be taken according to the instructions. Regular aromatherapy massages or reflexology assist the body to unwind and let go of tension. Essential oils of lavender, neroli, bergamot, clary sage, ylang ylang, and sandalwood are valuable used in the bath or a burner.

Nosebleeds

First, lie down. When the bleeding slows and you can manage it, take two small cotton balls and soak them in ice-cold water to which 2 drops of essential oil of lemon have been added. Gently insert a ball in each nostril. Placing a cold compress with lavender on the back of the neck will also help. Once the bleeding has stopped, use a cold compress of witch hazel to keep the area cool and reduce any inflammation. If the patient is in shock, they should be given Rescue Remedy and arnica.

Rheumatism and arthritis

The painful, inflamed joints that are caused by rheumatism and arthritis can be soothed with herbal remedies—but it is strongly advised to visit a qualified medical herbalist who can fully assess the situation in depth and prescribe treatment

accordingly. Dietary advice should also be sought because certain foods can aggravate rheumatism and arthritis. Devil's claw (*Harpagophytum procumbens*) is very effective for some people, and should be tried for a month. If there is no improvement, discontinue and try another remedy. Either

and baths, all using essential oils, can help. The best oils are lavender, marjoram, rosemary, and chamomile.

Shock

Rescue Remedy and arnica are the first remedies to take after shock. Essential oil of neroli, peppermint, or lavender should be sprinkled on a tissue and given to the patient to sniff repeatedly. Make sure the patient takes enough time to recuperate, sitting and resting or lying down if possible for half an hour. Do not allow someone suffering from shock to drive or engage in strenuous activity immediately afterward. Sometimes the symptoms of shock are delayed and it is important to allow enough time for this.

buy proprietary herbal tablets of devil's claw, or make a tincture and take 5–10 drops diluted in hot water three times a day. Devil's claw can be successfully combined with meadowsweet. The supplement glucosamine is particularly recommended, especially if Devil's claw doesn't work. Hot compresses, gentle local massage to the affected area,

Sinusitis

The best remedy is regular steam inhalation with essential oils of either lavender, tea tree, benzoin, thyme, eucalyptus, peppermint, or pine. These all help to clear the head and sinus, relieving headaches and pain around the eyes and face. The homeopathic remedy Natrum muriaticum may also help.

Slivers (Splinters)

Sometimes these can be very difficult to remove—and painful if removed with tweezers! Soak the affected part of the body in some hot water to which 2 or 3 drops of bergamot essential oil have been added. The oil should draw the sliver (splinter) out of the skin. If this does not work and it remains embedded, use a proprietary herbal drawing ointment that contains marshmallow and slippery elm. Once the sliver (splinter) is out, dab a drop of lavender oil on the wound to ensure that it does not become infected.

Sprains and strains

Apply cold compresses of witch hazel, or essential oils of lavender or chamomile, to the affected area. Repeat until the swelling subsides a little and the initial level of pain has receded. Strap the joint lightly and gently to give it some support. Take arnica and Rescue Remedy to counteract any shock. The next day alternate hot and cold compresses, as above, to aid the healing process.

Stress

Stress is increasingly common in Western society. Stress, whether we know it or not, has a negative effect on our bodily systems, and impacts on digestion, the immune system, and blood pressure. Take some chamomile—in tea or as oil in a massage—to sooth and calm. Hop tea or an infusion of passionflower is good for anxiety (though don't use it if pregnant) and will also aid relaxation. Valarian can quiet an over-active mind and should be taken as a herbal infusion at night to aid rest

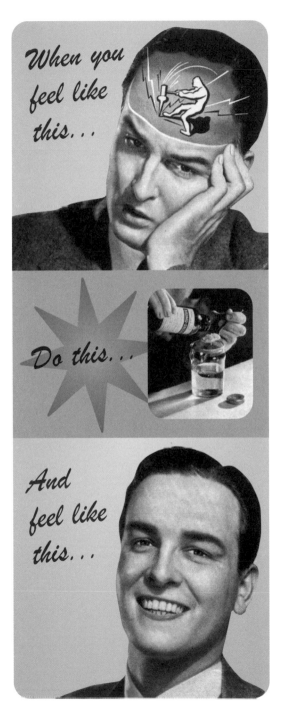

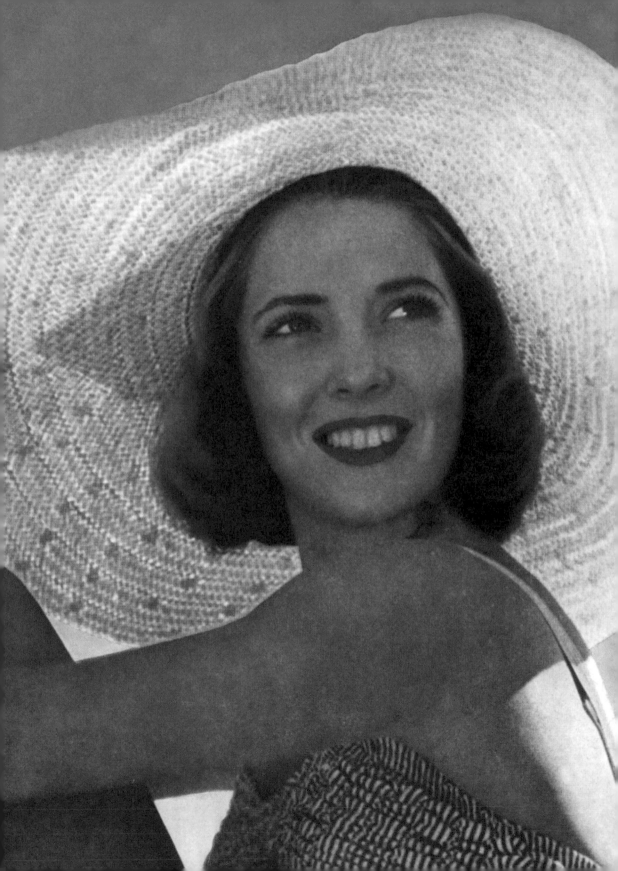

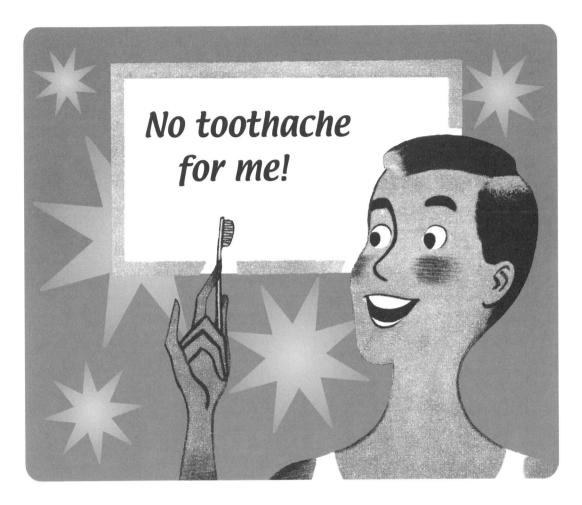

and sleep (see also Insomnia). Be careful taking Valarian during the day because it may cause tiredness. Avoid all sorts of caffeine.

Sunburn

Moderation in sunbathing is the best policy; the best rule is to expose yourself to less sun than you think you can tolerate. Always remember to use the correct sun screen factor for your skin type, and remember to reapply it frequently especially after swimming.

Cover your head and drink as much water as you can. A sunburn comes on gradually, and if you notice you are going pink while still lying in the sun, you are likely to have painful sunburn some hours later. As soon as the discomfort of red, sore skin appears, take a cool bath with 6 drops of chamomile essential oil. Apply generous quantities of After Sun lotion as soon as you are dry. This will be absorbed quickly, so then apply the homemade After Sun lotion described in Chapter Five, and keep applying both lotions alternately once the previous application has been absorbed. If the redness and pain continue, apply a cold compress with lavender essential oil to the worst affected parts, and repeat until the skin has cooled down. Ensure that lots of herbal teas and water are drunk, and take homeopathic tablets of cantharis.

Toothaches

The best remedy for these are essential oil of cloves. Dip a cotton swab in clove oil and use this to gently rub all around the affected area. Then apply a hot compress with chamomile oil to the affected area of the face, and repeat once the first compress cools down. An alternative to clove oil is to make an infusion of sage or thyme and keep swilling this around the mouth using water that is as hot as you can bear.

Varicose veins

The classical, well-known herbal remedy for varicose veins is rutin, which is found in rose hips, blackcurrants, and especially buckwheat. Tablets called Rutivite™ are available, and these should be taken according to the instructions. The homeopathic remedy hamamelis may also help. A topical application of cypress essential oil—3 drops mixed into 1 teaspoon (5ml) of base lotion or almond oil—can be applied twice a day. Rest as much as possible keeping your legs elevated, and try sleeping with your feet propped up on a small pillow.

Warts and plantar warts (verrucas)

The homeopathic remedy thuja is recommended here. Another classic herbal treatment is to rub the milky juice from a dandelion stem onto the wart or planar wart (verruca). Once this dries into a thin film, repeat the application as often as you can. Eventually the wart will darken and fall off.

A poultice made of crushed garlic and fresh lemon juice can be left on verrucas overnight, but remember to wrap the foot in a plastic bag so the smell does not overwhelm you and impregnate your bedsheets. Alternatively a daily application of a single drop of essential oil or lemon or tea tree applied carefully with a cotton swab should cause the wart or plantar wart (verruca) to fall off in about a week.

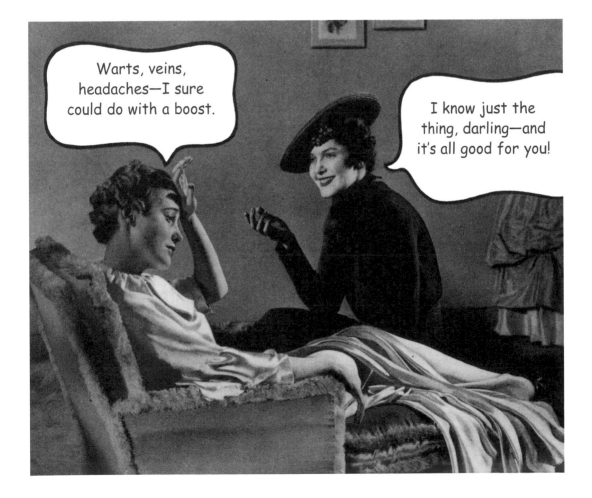

Index

Picture credits

All images below © Getty Images, Inc.
p. 3 Healthy and Glowing, 1932
p. 7 Steam Cabinet, 1960
p. 8 Leapfrog Ladies, 1941
p. 12 Health Foods, 1970
p. 17 Pick-Me-Up, 1961
p. 32 Preparing Food, 1941
p. 46 Medical Alternatives, 1946
p. 54 The Joy of Gardening, circa 1955
p. 98 The Answer's a Lemon, 1960
p. 101 Stretch Girl, circa 1965
p. 117 Practicing Yoga, circa 1940
p. 188 Modern Furnishing, 1953
p. 120 Self-examination, circa 1945

front cover (bottom left), p. 19, 20, 31, 37, 57, 59, 60, 63, 69, 79, 84, 90, 100, 112, 121, 129, 137, 134, 141 © Advertising Archive Ltd

p. 45 The Advertising Archive Ltd. / © SEPS: Curtis Publishing, Indianapolis, IN.

Important Note

The information and advice contained within this book are provided for reference and educational purposes only, and are not intended to diagnose, treat, cure, or prevent any specific disease or illness. The remedies are not specific to individual people or their particular circumstances and, as herbs and medicines can cause allergic reactions or unwanted side effects in some people, we suggest that you always use extreme caution when taking any natural remedy or other form of medication. Neither the author nor the publisher are medical professionals, and cannot accept responsibility, or be held liable, for anything that occurs as the result of the use, or misuse, of these remedies. Always consult a qualified medical professional if you have any concerns about your health and before you start any new health care regime.

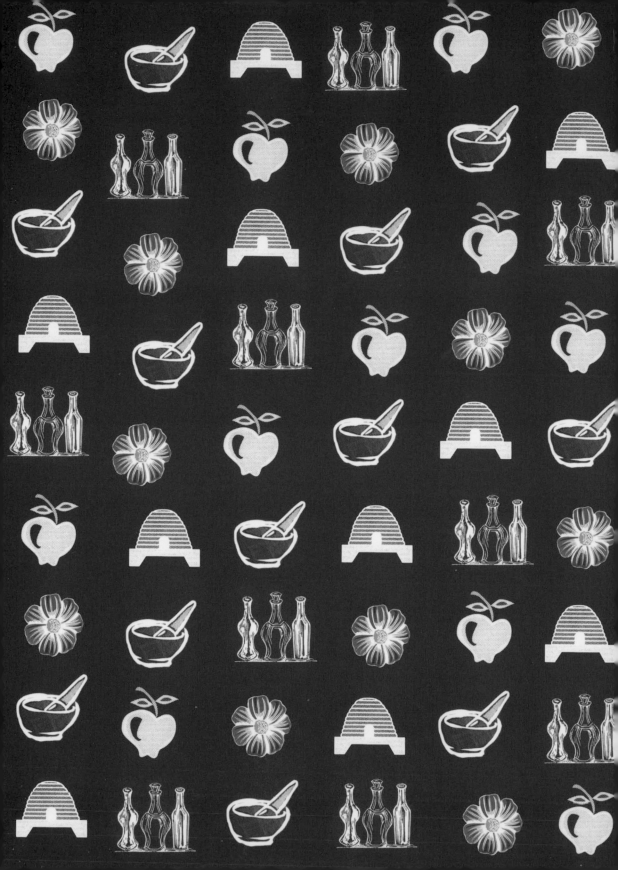